# Let the Patient Decide

# Let the Patient Decide

## A Doctor's Advice to Older Persons

Louis Shattuck Baer, M.D.

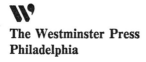

**The Westminster Press**
**Philadelphia**

*First edition*

Published by The Westminster Press®
Philadelphia, Pennsylvania

PRINTED IN THE UNITED STATES OF AMERICA

9 8 7 6 5 4 3 2

Grateful acknowledgment is made for the use of the poem from *As I Remember Him: The Biography of R. S.,* by Hans Zinsser. Copyright 1940 by Hans Zinsser. Used by permisssion of Little, Brown and Co. in association with The Atlantic Monthly Press.

R
726
.B23

**Library of Congress Cataloging in Publication Data**

Baer, Louis Shattuck, 1914–
  Let the patient decide.

  1. Terminal care—Moral and religious aspects.
2. Right to die. 3. Aged—Medical care. I. Title.
[DNLM: 1. Long term care—In old age—Popular works.
2. Attitude to death—Popular works. 3. Euthanasia—
Popular works. WT104.3 B141L]
R726.B23      174'.2      78-19014
ISBN 0-664-24207-3

**For Eve**
**who knows**

# Contents

# Foreword

If you are one of the 20,000,000 Americans over sixty-five, this book attempts to show you how to minimize your chances of ending your life in a nursing home and how you can prevent the medical prolongation of your act of dying.

I am a family doctor and have practiced medicine for forty years. In addition, since the end of World War II, I have had the learning experience of being on the faculty of a renowned medical school. In these four decades I have watched science make it increasingly hard for you or me to die a natural death in an American hospital. No matter how benevolent your doctor, he *dare* not let you "die in peace" in a hospital.

You could *suddenly* become too seriously ill to decide what you will and what you *will not* permit in the way of treatment. Your distraught family, acting in your behalf, will assuredly appeal to your doctors to do everything they can.

This may turn out well. Or it may result in medically staving off your death only to ensure lifeless years in an extended care facility.

The risks and unpredictable results in this common scenario

*are yours;* the decisions are made by others!

I am speaking not only about the heroic treatment of rare diseases but also of the *routine* measures used for the *common* serious illnesses of the seventh, eighth, and ninth decades of life.

These measures will surely include some if not most of the following:

1. Chemically balanced intravenous fluids

2. Powerful new antibiotics

3. Incredibly effective drugs and techniques to keep even the feeblest of hearts beating

4. Respiratory assistance measures of all types

5. Drugs to control fatal shock (very low blood pressure)

6. Renal dialysis to substitute for failed kidneys (even if you are eighty-five!)

7. And if all these measures fail to maintain, not your life, but your biological existence, and if finally your heart or breathing or both cease, then there will be mandatory attempts to resuscitate you. This list of routine measures is growing each year.

If, as my patients tell me, most people over sixty-five hope for a sudden death or a brief final illness, *why is this often denied them*—as it may be denied you—in an American hospital?

Part of the reason is that for ten thousand years doctors have seen themselves as death's opponents, a view also held by their patients. Doctors are not trained to take a passive role in the act of dying. They must avoid erring on the side of doing too little, and therefore they frequently, upon the insistence of the next of kin, do too much.

Up to ten years ago no medical schools taught a course on the art of dying. Beginnings are now being made, but it will take much time to influence the practice of medicine. The teachers will have to be our patients. This means that *you* have a contribution to make.

If you do not fear death but do dread "death in life," total invalidism, total dependence, and senility, you may well ask,

What can I do when my time comes to favor dying of natural causes in as short a time as possible?

The first part of this book is largely medical. It deals with specific cases indicating what happens to older patients in the intensive care unit, in the emergency room, and in the coronary care unit. You need to understand the great pressures that are on doctors and hospital staffs to treat all illnesses aggressively in order to decide what you want to happen to you. The later chapters deal with the possibilities that are open to you if you don't want your dying needlessly prolonged.

That is what this book is all about, for in actual practice the Right to Die laws and the Living Will are not enough!

The case histories and events are a composite picture.

I wish to thank my friend of twenty-five years, Miss Virginia Popplewell, for transmuting my pages of scribble and scratch into legible typography. I am also grateful to Pat Heemstra, Evelyn Szelenyi, Esther Fagin, and Meryem Agi for reams of "typing and retyping" done with enthusiasm and goodwill.

L.S.B.

# Part One
# The Dilemma

Please accept every assertion I make
as a question.

Niels Bohr, cited in Ruth Moore,
*Niels Bohr: The Man, His Science,*
*and the World They Changed*

# Chapter 1

## When You Neither Live Nor Die

Death offers man—the ordinary man—his last chance to
express his human potential to determine his own des-
tiny.

Robert M. Veatch,
*Death, Dying, and the Biological Revolution*

It is 4:15 P.M. on an August afternoon. Helen, my last
patient of the day, is sixty years old, married, and a retired
registered nurse. She has just returned from her eighth trip to
Los Angeles, where she has gone to visit her mother, who has
been confined to a nursing home for two years. Her husband,
Dan, and I were friends as undergraduates at the university.
They have been my patients for ten years.

Helen had asked my secretary to schedule a conference;
hence the late-afternoon appointment. I always save 4:15 to 5:15
for patients who "just want to talk" to me. At this time of
afternoon there is no rush. All the patients have been seen, and
a problem can be discussed leisurely and in depth.

I have practiced in this same office for thirty years. It is a
small, seventy-year-old cottage made into an office for two doctors. It has a large waiting room with a log-burning fireplace
that works!

Our bills are handwritten, we are not incorporated, we make

house calls, and we do not use collection agencies. We are open Saturday mornings. We are an endangered species—family doctors!

"It is just terrible, Dr. Baer!" Helen began. "My mother, who is eighty-six, was such a vital, active, and intelligent person. And now for two years she has not even known my name, or where she is, or who she is. She has difficulty swallowing and frequently chokes on her food even though it is liquid or pureed. The nurses spoon-feed her and bathe her. She has had a catheter in her bladder for one year, changed and irrigated at regular intervals. Every day they give her digitalis to strengthen her heart, a diuretic to get rid of the fluid, and an antibiotic to prevent infection.

"What really troubles me is that I know now my mother should never have had to spend these two years in a nursing home in the first place! It was those miserable I.V.'s [intravenous] they gave her in the hospital that did it. Without those she would have quickly died a natural death."

I encouraged Helen to give me all the details. She continued. "Mother had a stroke two years ago while living in her apartment. Dan and I were on vacation, and her own doctor was in Europe. It took two days for the hospital to reach me. I was told my mother was being cared for by the doctor who was on call for her personal physician. She had been in a coma since arriving on the intensive care unit, but they said that all her 'vital signs' were 'stable,' whatever that meant.

"My sixty-two-year-old unmarried sister was there and said she thought Mother was in the best hospital in Los Angeles. She said many residents and interns had examined Mother but she was not sure who was in charge of the case.

"When I arrived four days after Mother's admission she was still in a coma. From time to time antibiotics were injected into the I.V. tubing. The oxygen flow rate was adjusted.

"Thirty-six hours after landing in Los Angeles, I finally arranged to talk face-to-face with the doctor in charge. I think Dan helped by being rather peremptory with the secretary. I told the doctor I was an R.N. and asked him if he would transfer Mother from the intensive care unit to a private room, where I could help care for her. He answered that at present her condition was too precarious, the diagnosis too difficult, and her management too complicated to be handled elsewhere.

"I replied: 'My mother is an old lady with a bad heart, she has had a stroke, this is the fifth day she has been in a coma. Why can't she die in peace, with no tests, no oxygen, no antibiotics, and no intravenous?'

"His answer was that if I wanted to take charge of the case perhaps I would advise him whether or not burr holes should be drilled to rule out a subdural hemorrhage [a hemorrhage between the skull and the brain].

"I did not answer him but I seriously thought of taking Mother back to her apartment and caring for her myself. I wish now that I had.

"They did drill burr holes—there was no subdural hemorrhage. After a total of two weeks on the intensive care unit, receiving daily intravenous fluids, Mother slowly came out of her coma, but never recovered. She is left with what the Medicare diagnostic sheet calls 'Organic Brain Disease and Pseudo Bulbar Palsy,' due to a cerebral infarction. In plain language, she had a severe stroke which damaged the 'swallowing nerves' and destroyed the 'thinking' part of her brain. She can move her arms and legs but is uncoordinated and falls repeatedly.

"Why do the nurses now two years later continue to give her medicine? How much longer will it go on? What can I do to keep this from happening to me?"

"The first question is easy to answer," I said. "Her doctors know she will die if they stop any of those pills. As for how long it may all go on, I cannot say. Probably until your mother has a sudden fatal stroke or a fatal heart attack. As for your third question, 'How can you prevent yourself from spending two or three years in an extended care facility?' that is difficult to answer briefly. But it *is* a problem facing *you* and *me* and every other American who dreads being carried inadvertently beyond the winter's end of life by medical science and technology.

"If you don't want to end your life in a nursing home as your mother has, you must be absolutely *determined to do everything in your power to prevent this. It's not enough to wish this won't happen to you.* Rather, as Ibsen said, 'The will is all.'[1]

"You and I know there can be no infallible plan. But if you consider the usual chain of medical events that lead a patient to a nursing home, you can avoid the vast majority of them."

Helen looked at me questioningly. "What do you think are the most important causes? I would like to have some influence on the way death comes to me."

She took a notebook and a pen out of her handbag. I reached behind me and took down from my "philosophic therapy" library a volume entitled *Epicurus and His Philosophy.* From long use it opened to the page I wanted and I read to her Epicurus' famous dictum: " 'The only human freedom is to choose or to avoid.'[2] Epicurus enunciated that maxim twenty-three hundred years ago. He is speaking directly to you and your concern. To prevent ending your life in a so-called 'convalescent hospital,' you must use your freedom to choose and to avoid."

I went on. "Epicurus taught that some things happen of necessity—the immutable laws of cause and effect, for instance. Others happen by pure chance. Over neither of these can you exert any control. That sounds pretty final; not very much room to maneuver. But through your *freedom to choose and your freedom to avoid* any medical or surgical treatment, or any hazardous diagnostic test, you *do* have a real measure of control over the outcome of future medical events in your life.

"It is a fact that there are major differences in what *doctors* think are in their patients' best interests and what the *patient* may think."

I paused; Helen looked up at me from her notebook. "I'm not sure I see how that helps me."

"Let me try to be more specific. I agree with Robert Veatch that far too often today patients are 'losing freedom to a technocratic elite.'³ But in fact it is your right alone to choose what medical treatment you will accept and what you will avoid. Only you can decide when you wish to accept aggressive medical therapeutic treatment and when you wish to avoid this approach.

"It is also *your responsibility* to be sure that your doctor, as well as your family, knows what your wishes are. It is your responsibility to make them known in time, and your responsibility to make your decision while you have the health and vigor to make intelligent choices. You and Dan might read *Death, Dying, and the Biological Revolution* [our last quest for responsibility]. It is a good survey of the problem.

"As your doctor, I do not want my medical recommendation to be just what I may wish to try to accomplish for you. Rather, I want my advice to be based on what *you choose to have attempted* and on what *you want avoided.*"

Helen put down her pen, paused and said, "My decision would depend on the circumstances at the time."

"True enough. But as your doctor I need both general and specific instructions from you *before* a surgical emergency or a medical catastrophe occurs. Let me ask you: Since death is inevitable for all of us, have you thought of how you want to die? Would you eventually welcome a sudden, natural death or a brief final illness?"

"Absolutely!" she responded at once.

"Are you determined to do all you can to avoid ending your life as a senile and totally dependent invalid in a nursing home?"

"Certainly."

"In order eventually to have a natural death, would you be willing to forgo some of the treatments, tests, and operations that scientific and technical medicine can attempt—sometimes with benefit and sometimes with harm—to prolong your life and the function of your vital organs?"

She thought a while and then said, "Do you mean that to avoid three years in a nursing home, like my mother, I may someday have to choose to forgo a treatment or an operation that would conceivably prolong my life?"

"Precisely," I said, nodding.

She looked straight at me. "I would certainly choose to die a natural death rather than end up in a nursing home."

I picked up my pen and her record, saying, "I will remember what you have said and I will make a note to this effect in your chart now as a record of our conversation. Remember, you can always change your mind. The first person with whom you should discuss the matter is Dan."

We both stood up. As she was putting on her coat, I said: "Don't forget, you alone can decide to choose or to avoid any test or any treatment. I may have greater medical knowledge than you, but you have greater wisdom about yourself, your life, your hopes, your needs, and your desires."

As she turned to leave, Helen said: "It should be relatively simple for me to make up my mind about any major medical or surgical measure you might recommend for me.

"I would ask you: What are the chances it would cure me or greatly help me? What are the chances it could cause my death? What would be the major complications? What could happen with no treatment?"

"You are asking about the so-called 'risk/benefit ratio,' Helen. The problem is that most patients just weigh the chances of cure against those of death. They do not consider THE FOR-GOTTEN QUESTION which, after sixty-five, is crucial."

"What's that?"

"What are the chances that this measure, be it as simple as daily intravenous fluids or as hazardous as brain surgery or a total hip replacement, will neither kill me nor cure me, but will leave me in limbo, existing biologically but with my mind so damaged or my physical incapacity so great that I will be doomed to months or years in a nursing home?"

# Chapter 2

## The Yang and the Yin
## of Modern Medicine

> The intensivist has an obligation to ensure that there is no
> case in which the only "right" that remains to an inten-
> sive care patient is the right to utilize medical technology.
>
> Cynthia B. Cohen, Ph.D.,
> "Ethical Problems of Intensive Care,"
> *Anesthesiology,* Vol. 47 (1977)

The large electric clock on the bare wall says 0750. It is
plain, white, and circular, and it has black hands and a red
sweep second hand. It is located where it can be easily seen from
every part of this incredible room filled with nearly three quarters of a million dollars' worth of new scientific equipment,
much of it electronic.

Even the clock is scientific. One thirty A.M. is shown as 0130;
one thirty P.M. is 1330. Noon is 1200; midnight is 0000.

Where have I taken you? To the Naval Observatory at
Greenwich, England? Not at all! We are in an I.C.U. (intensive
care unit), probably the best place to observe the Yang (good
results) and the Yin (bad results) of modern American medicine.

The setting is a large Midwestern university hospital. It is a
world-famous teaching center. I am attending the annual meeting of a distinguished medical society. We are waiting for
"Grand Rounds" to begin in the intensive care unit.

You may have read that ancient Chinese cosmology taught that everything known to and experienced by human beings was composed of two principles: the Yang, which was positive and bright, and its opposite, the Yin, which was negative and dark. Combined, they produced all that comes to be. As we observe Grand Rounds today, we will see that this concept is just as true of the modern American hospital as it was of life in the Chang dynasty of China three thousand years ago.

I am convinced that today's scientific and technically oriented medical practice produces as many little-publicized and seldom-considered negative Yin results as it does the better-known positive Yang results.

Moreover, the older you are, the truer this dictum is. Today an American hospital has an equal ability inadvertently to prolong your death as it has the ability to relieve your suffering or restore your health.

I have no ax to grind. I'm not looking for any villains and I don't plan an exposé. I just want to examine the facts and clarify the problem so that those who are over sixty-five can better use their freedom to choose and to avoid certain kinds of medical care.

The questions at stake are fundamentally philosophical or ethical. That they arise in a medical setting should not lead anyone to conclude that they are the exclusive purview of the scientific expert. I agree with Robert Veatch when he states that the problems are "in but not of the realm of science," and that the questions these problems raise should be "patient-centered" rather than having, as Veatch concludes, "technology shift the bulk of the decision-making to those with technological expertise."[4]

We are standing in the holy of holies, a room where the twin gods Science and Technology are worshiped by the brightest young medical school graduates to be found in this country.

Here, on the intensive care unit, ACTION is the watchword. It usually has to precede reflection and frequently supersedes it. At 0800 the most important "devotional" gathering of the week will begin, Medical Grand Rounds!

The modern-day high priest of science, dressed in a pristine white laboratory coat, will enter this sanctum sanctorum surrounded by his acolytes. His title is Chief of Medicine. The Chief at this particular university hospital is the youngest man ever so appointed.

He is a vigorous, extremely brilliant man, age forty-one, who has spent his whole professional life in medical research and administration. He has published twenty-one papers on the chemistry of the blood, but he has never made a house call! No patient of his can ever call him directly at his home on weekends or at night. He does not attend any patient in any nursing home. He does not see patients in the emergency room at 1:30 A.M. but on the ward the next day when the case has been "worked up" by the resident. He has missed the learning experience of these activities and of always being available to the patient and the patient's family. Nevertheless, he can choose his acolytes from the top 10 percent of the graduating classes of our finest medical schools. They worship him!

The room we are in has been newly remodeled and is the most modern intensive care unit within a hundred-mile radius. The tabernacle around which we will soon gather is the bed of the first patient whose case is to be presented.


## GRAND ROUNDS BEGIN

At exactly 0800 the Chief of Medicine, attended by his senior resident, two assistant residents, and two interns, enters the intensive care unit. I stand with twenty-five visiting doctors in a semicircle at the foot of Bed One.

Today's cases are ones that exemplify blood chemistry and

nutritional problems. All the patients have grave difficulties with eating, drinking, swallowing, digestion, or the excretion of waste matter. The scientific problem of each case is presented lucidly by the intern.

The assistant resident describes the treatment being given the patient. The senior resident gives a brief report of the general results of this treatment at this particular hospital. Finally, the Chief makes comments based on his experience.

There were six cases. Fifteen minutes per case. All remarks were brief and scientific. Rounds were over at 0930. One and a half hours of pure science and technology!

After rounds, I stay on to go over the charts in detail at leisure. As a family doctor, I know there are *nonscientific* aspects of these cases which I wish to examine.

Before sitting down at the nursing station to review the charts of the six "cases" (the usual terminology on Grand Rounds is "this case" demonstrates thus and so, *not* "this patient" or "this sick person" demonstrates thus and so), I walk into the nurses lounge to have a cup of coffee. There are perhaps six nurses in the room and several more come and go while I am there. There is a big cake cut for a nurse who is retiring after twenty years of service at this hospital, five of them on the intensive care unit.

I am standing bent forward to draw my cup of coffee from the percolator. My Medic-Alert bracelet is clearly visible around my left wrist.

"Might I ask you why you wear that bracelet, doctor?" said the nurse who was retiring.

I show it to her.

"Do you mind if I read it out loud to the other nurses?"

"Not at all."

She reads: "Positively no resuscitation, no I.V., no injection, no intubation!"

By way of explanation I say, addressing all the nurses in the lounge: "At my age, when my time comes, I want 'to go'! No heroic measures for me, or for my wife. You could not get either of us on your splendid intensive care unit if we had a purely medical problem."

There was a chorus of "Me, too!" "Boy, I agree!" "You said it!" "Right on, Dr. Baer!"

It was interesting to hear the sentiment of nurses who care for the patients *eight hours every day*. They probably know the feelings of patients and families better than most.

Let us now review the descriptions of the patients who were presented at this conference. It is hoped that they will help you to draw your own conclusions, or at least be prepared to ask some new questions of yourself and of your doctor regarding the good and ill effects of modern medicine for some older patients with chiefly medical problems.

The first patient was pure Yang. A thirty-four-year-old policeman with multiple gunshot wounds of the abdomen had not been able to eat for ten days. He had been kept in perfect nutritional and chemical balance by a skillful administration of intravenous fluids of varying types monitored daily by computerized, automated chemical analyses. His bowels remained totally at rest while his wounds healed. His life was saved and he will shortly be back working as vigorously as ever.

The second patient illustrated how the hoped-for Yang results often end in months or years of increasing Yin. She was a sixty-eight-year-old woman who for twenty years had had a slowly progressing disease of the kidneys. Twenty years ago such a disease always ended in uremic poisoning and death. However, she had been coming to the hospital for life-prolonging dialysis treatments three times weekly for the past two years. She is now worn out by the ordeal, as is her family. She no longer has strength or stamina, and is totally dependent on her husband, grown children, friends, and neighbors for assistance the four days she is at home. She weighed 83 pounds when we saw her.

I noticed a note written by the social service worker assigned to this case. The patient is quoted as saying that if she had known two years ago what she and her family were to suffer, she would never have started the dialysis program. Two years of suffering, losing ground every month, have obviously taught this patient that a relatively quick, painless death—most of it spent in a sleep, stupor, or a deep coma—would have been far better at her age for herself and her family.

Younger patients who are otherwise in good health are given an extra lease on life with dialysis while they are hopefully awaiting a kidney transplant. But many patients over age sixty-five have only the act of dying prolonged. This patient clearly illustrated technical perfection on Grand Rounds. All her blood chemistry, blood electrolytes, and blood gases were normal. In spite of this I believe she demonstrates how overwhelming the Yin effects can be, even when all the scientific criteria are satisfied. I learned two months after the Grand Rounds that the patient refused to return to the hospital and died quietly at home in eight days.

Most of us want to live a full life, but not at *any* cost! And unfortunately we can no longer leave every decision to the doctor. A large number of younger specialists are so captivated by the possible Yang results of medical technology that they tend to minimize the ever-present Yin possibilities which you, as the patient, can only disregard at your great peril. In fact, the Yin side of medicine is often a direct route to years of diapered and poseyed (a posey belt is a restraint to prevent falling) incompetence in a "convalescent hospital." The only trouble is that 95 percent of "convalescent hospital" patients don't "convalesce." I think that older patients need much more exposure to the possible consequences of the Yin side of modern medicine than is generally available today.

I recall many articles in the past twenty-five years extolling the Yang side of American medicine. The triumphs have been made familiar to all by the press and television. But I do not remember many feature articles or television programs depicting the dark Yin side.

The list is just as long, but the public is less familiar with it. I recently heard an intensive care unit nurse with several years' experience estimate that 90 percent of the *medical* (nonsurgical) patients over sixty-five years of age who are admitted to the intensive care unit are done more harm than good. My estimate is 80 percent Yin, 20 percent Yang! The intensive care unit is a fertile place to see both sides of the picture.

The third patient appeared to be pure, undiluted Yin. He is a prime example of technology and science and its lack of humanism.

The man was seventy-two years old and a "perfect case" for presention at Grand Rounds to a distinguished group of "visiting firemen." He had the great misfortune to be dying of a rare and interesting disease just when a new, highly technical, heroic, and ultrascientific treatment became available. This treatment has saved some lives, usually younger people (Yang result), but has prolonged the act of dying in many others (Yin result). It is called total parenteral hyperalimentation, which I will explain.

The patient presented at Grand Rounds had severe cirrhosis of the liver, secondary to a rare disease called hemosiderosis. In this disease, for some unknown reason large amounts of iron are deposited in the liver and cause much scarring and destruction of the liver cells. Death comes slowly when the liver finally can no longer carry out its main function, which is that of changing the food we eat into chemicals suitable to circulate in the blood.

Parenteral hyperalimentation, introduced about 1971, is used when a patient for any cause cannot eat or digest food for many days or several weeks. The patient eats nothing and is put on pure protein, carbohydrates, and fats, which is given intravenously through a tube passed into the jugular vein. These foods have been suitably prepared by the chemists so that they can nourish the body without passing through the liver or the digestive tract. A patient can be nourished for many weeks without any liver, stomach, or intestinal function whatsoever. He can even gain weight!

This patient had been in and out of this particular teaching hospital half a dozen times in the past four years, usually for severe gastrointestinal hemorrhage caused by the advancing cirrhosis of his liver. All these episodes were treated with multiple blood transfusions.

At age sixty he had been a strong and vigorous man weighing 190 pounds, all muscle! Now he weighed 115, and was dying. His present admission was not for another hemorrhage. Rather, it was a total liver failure due to the destruction of his liver cells. He was deeply jaundiced and mentally confused. In far-advanced disease of any *vital* organ, the mind naturally is affected and thinking impaired.

For five weeks on the intensive care unit, he had been kept alive with intravenous fluids containing pretreated fats, carbohydrates, and protein. That is to say, total parenteral nutrition.

His case was presented with multiple graphs to show the exquisite perfection of his blood chemistry and his blood gases. A metabolic tour de force, illustrating the newest advance in modern medicine! He had had no food for thirty-five days of this spectacular treatment . . . or was it treatment?

A not infrequent complication of this treatment is sepsis with high fever, requiring antibiotics intravenously and the removal of the catheter in the jugular vein and its surgical replacement. This happened twice to this patient.

He had no family, and because of the advance liver failure his mind was dulled. He did not have the understanding or strength to discuss his case or request termination of the treatment. The only justification for using this latest scientific development for this incurable patient seemed to me that of giving the younger doctors practice with a new technique. This patient died after ten months in a nursing home.

The fourth patient was again a Yang result. A young man whose liver and bowel had been severely damaged in a motorcycle accident was kept alive by total parenteral nutrition while the necessary surgical measures were taken that eventually returned him to his home in good health. The treatment kept him alive for a period of six weeks, but because of his youth he had a Yang result. Heroic measures for the young and strong have a much higher percentage of Yang results. Heroic measures for those in their seventh, eighth, or ninth decade often lead to more Yin results.

The fifth patient also exemplified, in my opinion, poor Yin medicine. She was presented to demonstrate the treatment of dehydration and malnutrition. She had such far-advanced progressive Parkinsonism (uncontrolled shaking of hands and head), that she was a total invalid. She was seventy-eight years old and had been cared for at home by her husband, who was also seventy-eight. He had spoon-fed her for over a year, took her to the bathroom in a wheelchair, and, with the aid of the visiting nurse, had kept her clean and comfortable.

The drugs she took to help in some measure alleviate the muscle spasm of her arms and legs and head had by now affected her thinking and her ability to swallow.

The day before Grand Rounds she was admitted to the intensive care unit, semi-stuporous. Yet the aggressive Chief Resident ordered the full battery of blood and laboratory tests and constant intravenous feedings and fluids to correct her dehydration.

This he accomplished. Her case was presented. It was scientifically perfect, so that instead of peacefully dying a few hours after admission and not regaining consciousness from the stupor, she was rehydrated. Two days after Grand Rounds she was transferred to a nursing home, where she continued to exist, being fed through a nasal gastric tube (a tube passed through the nose into the stomach) for six more months. Surely this is a Yin result. The treatment produced much needless suffering for the patient and her husband, all in the name of science and so-called "good medical care."

The final case appalled us! A seventy-two-year-old man with inoperable cancer of the stomach which had already spread to the liver weighed 81 pounds on admission to the intensive care unit. When he was presented to us after four weeks of total parenternal hyperalimentation he had gained 13 pounds. The Chief enthusiastically explained that the purpose of the treatment was to "build the patient up" so that he would be strong enough to have chemotherapy (chemical treatment of his cancer) and radiation!

## GRAND ROUNDS EVALUATED

Here we have seen technical medicine at its perfection.

In my candid judgment, except for the policeman and the motorcyclist, the other patients were mistreated. From the small group of patients we saw, it is clear that young and middle-aged patients whose chief problems are surgical benefit greatly from a modern intensive care unit. But it seems that patients over sixty-five suffering from serious medical complications of chronic illnesses are apt to be done a great disservice by the aggressive and heroic treatment available in an intensive care unit.

Persons over sixty-five may well someday have to choose death from natural causes to prevent months or years of existence in a nursing home after "successful, lifesaving" measures on an intensive care unit. You can't gamble on achieving the

Yang without risking the Yin! Most patients of any age are willing to risk death in the hope of curing a grave disease. They forget the possible "third side of the coin"—the Yin, not of death but of years of nonliving, total dependency, and senility.

Later, on the plane back to San Francisco, I found myself seated beside a colleague, also in his seventh decade of life.

I purposely engaged him in conversation. "What did you think of Grand Rounds?"

His reply was forceful and immediate. "They would not get me in their intensive care unit as a medical patient! It may be great for the young or vigorous middle-aged, and I might go there for a day or so postoperative or after a bad car accident. But if I have a serious medical problem, I want a private room with an old-fashioned nurse who will wash my face with a cool cloth, rub my back at night, give me ice chips to suck if I'm thirsty, and even hold my hand if I'm apprehensive! If she wants to check my pulse, she will feel my wrist and not read the rate off the electronic telemeter at the nursing station down the hall!"

I nodded. "I guess we feel the same way, but I am sure most of the members of our medical society who are twenty-five years younger than we are would disagree."

"You're right. Of course they would disagree. They aren't old enough to have suffered long and deeply themselves. They have just *seen* suffering and prescribed for suffering, but have not really felt it in their bowels."

He ended our discussion with some remarks which went about like this:

"We internists and family doctors have to help our patients regain control over what happens to them near the end of their lives. I believe we must teach them the real danger of both prolonging and increasing the suffering that can come from overenthusiastic applications of technology to the treatment of any chronic or serious medical problem they may have. It is, after all, their body, and they now have to make it their responsibility!"

To that I replied, "We must emphasize the Yin side of medicine for some patients over sixty-five."

My friend was Chinese. He understood what I meant!

# Chapter 3

## It's Difficult to Die in America

> The tide of technical revolution in this atomic age can so captivate, bewitch, dazzle and beguile us that calculative thinking may someday come to be accepted and practiced as the only way of thinking. *The issue is keeping meditative thinking alive.*
>
> Martin Heidegger, *Discourse on Thinking*

As late as 1831, the British Navy still used the hourglass at sea! Since that time there has been a veritable explosion of scientific knowledge, much of it in the field of medicine and health care. More than a thousand articles are published each month describing ways that modern medicine deals with disease and disability, and extends life. Polio and tuberculosis have virtually disappeared; radioactive iodine effectively treats toxic goiter; drugs can control serious depression or manic agitation; hip joints and diseased arteries can be replaced; artificial valves can correct the malfunctioning heart; the triumphs of eye surgery are nearly incredible; the transplant of whole vital organs (such as the kidneys) has produced amazing results. These and many more of the positive achievements of medical science and technology are widely reported and generally known. But there may be only one article published per month about how to make death easier.

## SCIENCE AND TECHNOLOGY DOMINATE

Premedical students are chosen from the brightest scientific minds in this country. The final applicants to medical school are tested and retested to ascertain their scientific acumen. Their high school records are studied and restudied. Their college performance is scrutinized carefully to be sure that all students admitted to the medical school are in the top 3 percent insofar as their scientific aptitude is concerned. But whether they will be compassionate or whether their practice of medicine will focus primarily on what is in the best interests of the patient we have no means of evaluating at the time a student is selected to enter medical school.

Medical students in the United States have so much to learn in the areas of science and technology that the liberal arts are virtually crowded out of their education. Roland Stevens, Clinical Associate Professor of Surgery, University of Rochester Medical School, phrased it well when he said: "Teaching in medical schools has now for more than two generations been in the hands of a group not noted for their contribution to humane letters. For the most part, indeed they are wholly innocent of such matters."[5]

Writing about those physicians chosen to staff our medical schools, Alexander Rush, Associate Professor of Clinical Medicine, University of Pennsylvania School of Medicine, had this to say:

> To these new leaders fell the responsibility of training a new generation of young physicians. . . .
>
> The direction of their efforts was toward the production of graduates steeped in the basic sciences and nurtured to become faculty and hospital-based specialists.
>
> Emphasis became centered upon disease and what modern scientific technology might be able to do about it, not upon the unfortunate being afflicted with the disease.

Recent graduates in medicine possess an awesome knowledge of the basic pathophysiology of disease coupled with supreme confidence in the ability of medical technology to solve all problems. What they lack is a compassionate approach to the patient.[6]

Small wonder that doctors are science-oriented.

*American hospitals and their staffs are geared to save your life at any cost!* Hospital administrators and boards of directors, in an effort to make their hospital the most advanced in the area, supply the medical staff with much appallingly expensive new scientific equipment every year.

That all has to be paid for, it has to be used—and I am sure it is often the patient who pays.

I have never seen a course in medical school entitled "Selective Limitation of Therapeutic Measures," although the Critical Care Committee of the Massachusetts General Hospital now advocates this for some of its patients. The problem is that the most important impetus for change *must* come from the patient, not from doctors or "optimal care committees." Most patients do not feel competent to take such initiatives.

The way serious illness in an older patient is usually managed today is well described by Martin G. Netsky, a doctor whose mother was a patient.

The system, confronted by the body within its halls, was put inexorably in motion. . . . They had been taught that life must be saved at all costs and at all times. . . . They paid no heed, however, to the wishes of the living, nor of the almost dead, but only to their own presumptions.[7]

It seems that sometimes on an intensive care unit the purpose is to utilize the machines. None of this expensive equipment is there to make dying in the hospital any easier. Simple morphine will do that! All these powerful drugs and the technically com-

plicated apparatus, although helpful for the seriously ill young
and middle-aged, make dying a natural death for the patient
over sixty-five much harder, much longer, and much more expensive.

American medicine for the past seventy-five years has become world famous for its scientific technical expertise. This has
produced many thousands of medical and surgical "miracles."
But this same emphasis on using science to cure has produced
a steady stream of thousands of patients in the seventh, eighth,
or ninth decade of life who were saved by science only to end
up in a convalescent hospital. They stay three days in the intensive care unit, ten days in a hospital room, and ten months to
three years in a nursing home.

A means must be found to free the patient from the tyranny
of a technological (or bureaucratic-professional) imperative to
keep him or her alive at all costs. In reality, all these scientific,
frequently painful and risky tests and treatments, which may be
done with the best of intentions, often simply exchange one fatal
disease for another.

Moreover, *nursing homes too are geared to keep the senile
patient's existence going on and on.* Although 90 percent of their
patients are incurable, many nursing homes now have patient
charts similar to those in the acute hospital, and their pharma-
cies have access to every life-prolonging drug available to an
intensive care unit.

The slightest sign that Mrs. J. has a cough and fever, or Mr.
G. is short of breath and his chest sounds congested, or Mrs. L.
is losing weight, or Miss B. has a urinary tract infection, brings
a telephone call to the attending physician. About nine tenths
of the time, the scientifically correct medicine is ordered by the
patient's doctor. Natural death is again denied to the senile
patient who has not been able to name the month of the year
or the day of the week since admission. I call this "Unloving
Care,"[8] for I know from forty years of practice as a family

doctor that *death* rather than continued medicated existence is the *summum bonum* of these patients.

A nursing home is not a boarding home! In the latter there are no built-in, life-sustaining techniques; no charts are kept. The elderly in a boarding home are more independent and more alert than the average patient in a nursing home. They *live;* the nursing home patient *exists.* Your doctor has to certify that you are capable of self-care and require no nursing before a boarding home will accept you as a "resident" (not as a "patient").

I wish strongly to emphasize that the nursing home personnel are among the hardest-working and most underpaid in the whole health care profession. It is not they that I challenge, but something more subtle and nebulous. It is the ascendancy of science in institutions where simple humanity alone should prevail. The staffs I know are devoted to helping their helpless charges, but other priorities frequently make their task an exercise in futility.

## A PREVAILING ASSUMPTION ABOUT LIFE

In addition to advances in science and technology, there are social factors that make dying difficult. Since Cro-Magnon man did his paintings in the Lascaux Cave, life has been thought to be the greatest gift of the Creator. Individuals have so regarded it, religion has stated it, and society as a whole has found this to be true. Therefore it is widely believed that *life must always be preserved.*

The trouble is that social mores and our thinking as a race has lagged far behind the extraordinary advances of medical science in the past hundred years.

None of my patients over sixty-five consider permanent confinement to a nursing home a gift to be desired. They dread it and want above everything else to avoid it and to have me help them avoid it. Still, it is hard to change the widespread ethical belief that human life must be sustained at all costs. The growing demand for the opportunity to die without existence-prolonging medical measures still has to face the deep-rooted, instinctive desire of the health team to sustain the function of the vital organs to the end and in the case of the heart and lungs to restart them once they have failed.

## FAMILIES DEMAND EVERYTHING POSSIBLE

As a family doctor, I have often found that the greatest social pressures on me to continue existence-sustaining measures in a patient come from the patient's family. When an emergency medical problem, such as a severe stroke in a previously healthy parent, suddenly confronts the grown "children," they will insist that "everything possible be done" for their mother or that "the finest specialist" be called in to save their father.

Any hint from the doctor that it might be better to relax and let matters take their course is not well received unless such a possibility has been carefully discussed by the patient and the family before it occurs. That does not take place as often as it should. It is the exception, not the rule.

With the hundredfold increase in the ability of medical science to prolong biologic existence, frequently by very simple measures, adult "children" have to learn to let their parents "go." A wife or a husband must now learn to make it easier for a doctor to help the mate, by doing *less* medically rather than by doing *more*. When some member over sixty-five can no longer communicate and is confronted by the possibility of years of total invalidism and dependence, too few families consider carefully enough what that person's wishes would be in such circumstances. So the doctor is asked: Is there a chance he will live? Will she speak? The chance may be less than one in a thousand, but the family clings to it. The intravenous with its antibiotics drips on, and a death from natural causes (a stroke, for example) that would have come quickly in three to five days with just good nursing care *is transformed into three years in a nursing home,* by the well-intentioned, simple but *so* effective medical measures that have been used.

The dilemma is difficult in the extreme for the doctor and the family. But it won't fade away. It must be discussed widely by all older citizens. If more people discuss this problem well in advance, doctors and families can find a better approach than we have so far. For the next of kin of a stuporous or comatose patient to say, "Do everything you can and if that fails I pray the Lord will take him," or "I can't play God," may well lead away from *life* and ensure years of NONLIVING in a nursing home for the patient.

Many a devoted, loving wife has unwittingly committed an "unloving act." Sensing by instinct, after her husband has suffered a devastating stroke, that he may not recover the power of speech or reason and will indeed have to be permanently confined to a nursing home for care, she will say to the doctor, "I would never be able to live with myself if you did not do everything you could to save his life." So on and on goes the I.V. Eventually, the helpless patient becomes able carefully to swallow a liquid or soft diet and so is doomed by "loving kindness" to two to three years, on an extended care facility, to DEATH IN LIFE.

These needless, sad, and tragic outcomes could be prevented by facing in advance the ever-present possibility of the always unexpected illness or injury which makes communication impossible at the time the disaster strikes.


### THE NOT SO GOOD SAMARITAN

The widow or widower living alone with no family nearby faces a special risk. If he, or more frequently she, is taken suddenly seriously ill, neighbors or friends will call the ubiquitous emergency ambulance service. The patient will be whisked willy-nilly to the nearest emergency room, there to begin the whole chain of events which are designed to prevent a quick death but which often only produce prolonged invalidism and institutionalization.

We need some restraint to forestall the automatic triggering of this modern version of the good Samaritan. Medical and surgical expertise often saves the lives of the young and the healthy middle-aged, but frequently ends in disaster for the person who is advanced in years.

The restraint has to be initiated by the patient before the crisis! Stone Age man had his prescribed tribal death rituals, so did each successive ancient civilization, so do all organized religions. In like manner, so does science and technology in late-twentieth-century America. Today in this country it seems that no one in an urban area, not even the elderly, can be treated with ordinary goodwill at work with reason. No one, it appears, can die without the thirty-minute American Heart Association's "approved" attempt at resuscitation.

## OTHER SOCIAL FACTORS

Today we live in smaller and smaller quarters. There is no room for a sick or dying member of the family. Families are smaller; frequently, in urban areas, husband and wife both work. The children are in school and have part-time jobs. There is no one at home to care for an invalid.

Money is also a factor. My years in medical practice convince me that a patient with a large fortune is apt to have too much medical care. A notable exception was Charles Lindbergh, who was able to take firm control over the way he wished to die. The same seems to me to be true of the very poor. When medical care is entirely supported by tax dollars, there is much more treatment than might occur otherwise. Doctors tend to order more tests and X-rays and institute more therapeutic procedures when they do not have to consider whether the patient's hospital bill will be paid. From what I have observed, none of these tests makes dying easier.

Actually, the older patient in large county or Veterans Administration hospitals is a source of many articles on the newest, most expensive, and the most technically sophisticated means for prolonging existence in the chronically ill. The medical literature of the past thirty years confirms this observation. These are but a few of the factors that make it difficult to die in America.

# Chapter 4

## Doctors Don't Always Know Best

I am going to make one suggestion regarding terminology,
that we do not use the term "life" except to refer to the
total personal being—Body, Mind, and Spirit.

> Henry P. Van Dusen, Opening Remarks,
> First Euthanasia Conference,
> Nov. 23, 1968

### DOES THE DOCTOR ALWAYS KNOW BEST?

"I must be getting old, Lou," my friend the radiologist re-
marked. "All the younger doctors seem to be such activists, even
with older patients. They are right there pushing every test and
using every new instrument and "scope" the cornucopia pours
out. For the older patients this may occasionally be beneficent,
but from what I have seen, inadvertently and not infrequently
it is maleficent."

The concern my friend raised is one I share. My convictions
about the effects of aggressive medicine on older patients are
clear and firm. But in all honesty, it must be said that they do
not reflect the views of many of my colleagues. Moreover, the
issues are too complex to yield to simple solutions, particularly
solutions that would make the doctors the villains of the script.

Without doubt, the doctor has a significant role to play in our
effort to avoid dying in a nursing home. We need to understand

his philosophy, and also some of the pressures that move him to do the things he does in treating patients.

## KNOW YOUR DOCTOR'S PHILOSOPHY

If your doctor's philosophy is to ward off death as long as possible, his judgment will lead him to use science and technology aggressively. If you survive a catastrophic illness but only as a permanent and total invalid, your doctor nevertheless has done everything possible. Too late then to ask if he did too much. His treatment was consistent with his philosophy. He did what he believed he should have done.

But we are speaking of your life or your death, your mode of living or dying! It *must* be *your* judgment that ultimately prevails. To achieve this you have to crystallize a philosophy *now* while you are well. Then you must unequivocally make known to your doctor what you CHOOSE and what you wish to AVOID from scientific medicine. In the rare circumstance that your doctor's philosophy in such that he cannot agree with you, ask him what he advises. But remember that today the initiative rests with you. If you do not come to an understanding with your doctor, the "scientific system" will take over—quite possibly to your great detriment.

## RAISE QUESTIONS WITH YOUR DOCTOR

Many older patients spend their last years in a nursing home because they and their families have assumed "the doctor always knows best." Helen, whom I introduced in Chapter 1, believed that doctors played a big role in what happened to her mother. Ever since the founding of Jericho, the physician has assumed a father figure. For millenniums he has acted and spoken in a paternalistic and authoritative way. Patients and their families say: "Do what the doctor advises," or, "The doctor told me to do such and such." The doctor has ordered (not asked) and the patient has said, "Thank you, doctor," and no questions asked.

But as Maria Huxley said, "No one knows best, for we all know differently."[9] Unless your doctor knows what you CHOOSE and what you wish to AVOID, he can by no means always know what is best for you.

Until 1900 we doctors could not prolong the act of dying of a senile or chronically ill patient. If anything, we always hastened the patient's death with our bleedings and purgatives and emetics. For thousands of years, saying "Yes, doctor" would *not* prevent your natural death. But in just the past seventy-five years (the practice lifetime of my father and myself), *all this has changed.* A simple, continuous intravenous drip can prevent natural death for days or even weeks.

If you are over sixty-five and are confronted with a serious medical or surgical problem, it is your RESPONSIBILITY to question your doctor closely as to the why of his recommendations. You *must* weigh your own desires, experience, and judgment equally with his medical opinion. Now more than ever before, you *must* make up *your* own mind whether or not to accept his recommendations. Medical paternalism was harmless and even served a purpose up to 1900, but it is all wrong in America in the late decades of this century.

## DOCTORS ARE HUMAN TOO

It is important, however, to try to understand the reasons why your doctor may be unwilling to let you die naturally without a "no holds barred" effort to keep your life going. A doctor may have strong personal, ethical, or religious reasons which urge him to action rather than inaction. He may find your threatened death a challenge to his personal power, his technical ability, and his intellectual capacity. The practice of medicine should be very humbling, but at the same time it *is* a supreme ego trip. When I graduated in 1938 all the nurses stood up when the doctor came to the nursing station! Literally, a senior nurse with thirty years of experience would rise when an intern of twenty-five would come to the desk. Our patients come to us as suppliants asking our help. The joke about God wanting to "play doctor" speaks to the point I am making.

Furthermore, we doctors are quite human. We experience all kinds of pressure and react to it! Peer pressure from colleagues on our own hospital staff to upgrade our knowledge and therapeutic acumen does not usually stimulate us to do less. It usually results in our doing more. Doctors don't "cotton" well to criticism and therefore are apt to try to stay a jump ahead rather than a step behind therapeutically. All this tends toward scientific medical intervention rather than just good nursing care and symptomatic treatment.

If your doctor's enthusiasm speaks more forcefully than his humility, your death may be *postponed,* but also your act of dying is apt to be *prolonged.* Sometimes this is good, but often, for the person over sixty-five, it is undesirable no matter how excellent it may appear in some abstract of one hundred cases published in a medical journal.

The question asked in a staff or clinical conference is usually, "Could this death have been prevented?" not, "Could this death have been made easier?" Or, "Could this life have been extended?" not, "Could the act of dying have been less prolonged?"

I have often noticed that *a doctor's age and health can profoundly influence his medical decisions.* If he is young, vigorous, strong, indefatigable, and has never suffered a prolonged or serious illness himself, he finds it hard to look on death as other than something to be defeated at all costs. The most enthusiastic interventionists I have seen in the intensive care unit are the doctors under forty.

If a doctor is in his later years of life and has experienced personally a major medical catastrophe, he is naturally much more apt to view his own death, or that of an older patient, more benignly. He is inclined to weigh the pros and cons of aggressively treating every threat to his older patient's life on a different scale than the young doctor. As Hilaire Belloc said in his biography of John Milton: "Good health draws a veil between a man and self-knowledge. Long-lasting health forbade him [meaning John Milton] contrition."[10]

Doctors have amazing skills and knowledge in certain areas, but they are human, they do make mistakes, and their wisdom does not extend to all the areas of life. Even in the arena of health care, particularly in the later years, we have seen that the doctor does not always know what is best for the patient.

Sometimes there are factors that exert pressure upon doctors to be more aggressive in the practice of medicine than a person may wish. It is well to understand what some of these pressures are.

## LEGAL FACTORS IN MEDICAL PRACTICE

There is an abundance of legal factors that tend to make *every doctor in this country practice defensive medicine.* Doctors order many more tests and more consultations than did the physicians practicing before World War II because physicians are conscious that every patient-doctor contact, be it even a telephone call, may lead to a million-dollar lawsuit. Malpractice premiums in some specialties and some states are more than $28,000 a year.

Some of this is our fault, some society's, some our patients', some the legal profession's. But whoever is to blame, we doctors are paying the premiums. One of the results is that at least 50 percent of the doctors routinely do and order *everything* possible to preserve life at *any* cost, so that at some future date a jury will not decide that the patient died because of the doctor's negligence. I recently saw a closed-circuit television program on cardiopulmonary resuscitation conducted by one of the most distinguished physicians in this country, Kevin M. McIntyre, M.D., J.D., Professor of Medicine at Harvard Medical School. It did not deal with *when* or *when not* to institute treatment, nor the basic or advanced life-support techniques; *it was on the medical-legal consequences of CPR!* You can well believe, if you are over sixty-five, that the legal profession makes it harder for you to die a natural death in America.

Another powerful factor affecting medical practice today is that the legal definition of death is not always clear. This adds to the doctor's dilemma. If for humane reasons we stop trying to save a patient's life before every criteria of death has been legally satisfied, we worry about a possible lawsuit.

There are now many definitions of death. It used to be simple. If you stopped breathing and your heart stopped beating, and your pupils dilated, you were dead. Not today!

You may have to have all these plus a flat electrocardiogram and flat electroencephalogram before you are pronounced officially dead.

Moreover, you may have to sustain one half hour of futile cardiopulmonary resuscitation before it is considered legally safe to pronounce you dead. Even if you are eighty or eighty-five, or even if chronic ill health has obviously sapped your strength and your will to live, it takes a great deal of fortitude for your doctor to pronounce you dead simply because your heart has stopped and your respirations have ceased.

While the malpractice lawyer looks figuratively over the doctor's shoulder, you will have your chest massaged, receive multiple electric shocks, have a tube placed in your windpipe, and your blood filled with half a dozen powerful intravenous medications, all to prevent a lawsuit!

Another legal problem concerns euthanasia. There are two

kinds, positive and negative euthanasia. The former I am *sure* is wrong. For a doctor to do something in a positive way to hasten the death of a dying patient is not ethical, is not good medicine, and is not allowed under any circumstances!

Negative euthanasia, which means doing nothing that will prevent natural death, is of course what I espouse. However, you can see for yourself that the differentiation is not always clear-cut. For example, when doctors order frequent, large (but nonlethal) doses of Demerol, a commonly used morphine derivative, or morphine to relieve the pain and apprehension of a patient dying of cancer, the patient as the result of the doctor's treatment sleeps more, eats and drinks less, and dies more quickly. This is *not* positive euthanasia, but it has that effect. I believe the law must begin to help us physicians *act positively in a negative fashion* so that we will not be obliged to delay natural death, *if this is what the patient desires.*

These are some of the legal factors with which the practicing physician must deal. Their effect is to encourage aggressive measures, even when they may not be in the best interests of the patient.


## GOVERNMENTAL PRESSURES

We doctors also experience much pressure from county, state, and federal government agencies who pay a large percentage of the bill for most patients over sixty-five. The federal government wants proof that we "come up to the mark," use the latest and newest techniques, take more and more courses in continued medical education so that we do not "miss a trick." The government gives us no bonus points for what we learn from our patients over a period of forty years! To count, it has to be a certified academic course approved for credit. But I have yet to see a course entitled "How to Keep Your Patient from Ending His Life in a Nursing Home."

## A MEDICAL SHIP WITHOUT A CAPTAIN

Another aspect of modern medicine that may not always serve your best interests has to do with the growing tendency toward subspecialization.

You will find today that often a seriously ill hospitalized patient with a complicated illness has no "captain of the medical ship."

A hundred years ago doctors tended to be whole-patient-oriented. Today, a large number of subspecialists are disease-oriented, or organ-oriented, or procedure-oriented. It is common for three specialists to make daily rounds on the same patient. One is interested in pulse and blood pressure and cardiac output. Another checks on the blood creatinine and urinary output. A third is concerned with vital capacity and blood gases, making sure that the bronchial tubes are clear. But perhaps no one knows or cares when the patient last had a bowel movement or if there was any time to sleep between the nonstop, twenty-four-hour-a-day tests and treatments. Such mundane matters are personal, not scientific problems.

I believe the older the hospitalized patient is, the more a family doctor is needed to say "enough is enough."

## A DOCTOR'S UNMEDICAL ADVICE
## TO OLDER PATIENTS

We have reviewed some of the factors that make modern medical practice aggressive in the treatment of all sorts of serious illnesses. We have shown that often in the case of older patients such practice may not be in their best interests. You may ask: "What can we do about it? Are we at the mercy of the medical establishment once we commit ourselves for medical care?"

One bit of practical advice is to be realistic in what you can expect from medical practice in our time. The thrilling advances in medical science and therapy over the last forty years have caused patients to expect too much. Many patients believe that all a doctor has to do is make the right diagnosis and apply the proper treatment and all will be well. Daniel Greenberg, writing in *The New England Journal of Medicine* for March 24, 1977, describes the American patient as "miracle-seeking."[11] If you are over sixty-five, the chances of finding a medical or surgical miracle are less, and the risk of disaster greater than when you are young or middle aged.

Don't press your doctor to do everything that can be done. There are too many instances in which the treatment is worse than the disease. Not a few patients are in nursing homes today as a result of strokes secondary to diagnostic tests or vascular surgery. All our efforts to reach a diagnosis or cure a disease can turn an ailment into a catastrophe. Ask what should reasonably be done rather than insist on *all* that can be done.

Talk over such possibilities with your doctor while you are able to do so. If you prefer a natural death to a lingering, incapacitating existence, tell him to forgo a possible medical or surgical miracle for the chance for you to die serenely with just good nursing care. The doctor is not likely to raise the issue with you, so it is your responsibility to raise it with him.

And finally, since you are the patient, you should give your doctor "strategic orders" for him to follow in case you are hospitalized for a serious illness. He then will issue "tactical orders" that conform to what you CHOOSE and what you wish to AVOID from modern scientific medicine.

## HOW DO YOU WANT TO DIE WHEN YOUR TIME COMES?

It is you patients alone who can teach your doctor *how you want to die.* Actually, there has been some research on this matter in Sweden. Gunnar Biorck, M.D., Fellow of the Royal College of Physicians, Stockholm, questioned a large number of people and concluded that "a majority of people want to die suddenly." Dr. Biorck concludes his article by asking: "Should sudden death be prevented in society at large? Or should we base our medical strategy on what people seem to wish?"[12]

For myself, I would consider a sudden death a great blessing. It is the one certain way to prevent me from becoming a senile invalid.

Ninety percent of my patients over sixty-five tell me the same thing.

# Chapter 5

## Death Preferred

Must all human beings admitted to an institution surrender to the conditioned reflexes of scientific team work?

Martin G. Netsky, M.D., "Dying
in a System of 'Good Care,'"
*The Pharos,* April 1976

My first emergency house call, more than thirty years ago, eventually ended with my patient going to a nursing home. It was probably this case which stimulated my concern about medicine's role in making problems worse than they need be.

The story concerns me, my patient, and my old chief of medicine. I had just recently opened my office in a suburb of San Francisco after four and a half years in the Navy Medical Corps during World War II. I had been out of uniform less than six months. The chief had befriended me, appointing me to a paid, part-time job with a faculty position and referring to me several private patients who lived nearby.

"My secretary said you called me, Baer, and wanted to talk about old Mrs. S., whom I referred to you."

"Yes, sir."

"What's the problem?"

"Well, sir, I saw her on an emergency house call at about 2:00 A.M. a couple of months ago and I've wondered ever since if I handled her case the way you would have."

I was thirty-two, the chief was sixty-three. He seemed to me but one step removed from Jehovah. He was universally admired by his patients and his colleagues. We younger staff physicians revered him for his erudition, humanity, and equanimity.

"I'll try to make it brief, Dr. C."

"Tell me the details, Baer. I no longer see patients on Friday afternoon and I'd rather sit here with you than tackle all the paper work that's waiting for me in my office."

"As you know, Mrs. Stone's daughter asked me to make a house call on her mother soon after you gave them my name. I did so and found the patient as you had described—an overweight, elderly lady. She said she was eighty-one, but her daughter told me she was eighty-six. She appeared comfortably cared for by her daughter and a part-time practical nurse.

"She had no particular complaints. I checked her medicines, which consisted of one tablet of digitalis daily, a laxative, some coated aspirin tablets, and Seconal for sleep. The chief nursing problem was that she was frequently incontinent and needed diapers at night to keep her dry.

"I saw her about once every two weeks. She was never dressed, because even with her daughter's help, this tired her too much. For the same reason she used a commode and was given a bed bath, as going to the bathroom or taking a regular bath was physically impossible. She never read. Her vision permitted her to read the headlines, but she did not understand their meaning. She was hard of hearing, but I could ask her questions by talking directly into her ear, which was fitted with a hearing aid.

"To test her acuity and acumen, one time I asked her to name the months of the year backward, starting with December. She totally failed. I asked her to name the last three Presidents of the United States. She could not. I tell you this to show you how much she had failed since you last saw her a year and a half ago."

The chief looked quizzically at me over the top of his old-fashioned Benjamin Franklin glasses. He raised his thick black eyebrows, which, in spite of his benign nature, gave him a rather Mephistophelian appearance. I thought he was indicating his desire that I get to the heart of the matter.

I continued. "The problem that is troubling me, sir, began at 2:00 A.M. on the Sunday in early January right in the middle of that three-day torrential rainstorm.

"Miss Stone called me directly at home [I give all my patients my unlisted telephone number], saying: 'Come quickly, Dr. Baer, I think Mother is dying. She is very short of breath.'

" 'Sit her up in a chair, keep her warm, and I'll be there in a few minutes.' Which I was, as house calls were easy to make on the Peninsula.

"As you can guess, sir, when I arrived it was immediately apparent that she had acute severe left ventricular failure, and, in addition, she had atrial fibrillation with a very rapid ventricular rate. [These terms mean failure of the heart's muscle to pump with sufficient strength and an abnormal, rapid, ineffective but not necessarily fatal rhythm.]

"I gave her intravenous aminophylline [to relieve her lung congestion], morphine [to relieve her shortness of breath], and intramuscular Mercuhydrin [to get rid of excess fluid]; and additional digitalis intramuscularly [to strengthen and slow the heart].

"Within minutes she was improved. I called an ambulance and had her taken to the hospital. There I continued full doses of all her medicines."

"Sounds like you handled it expertly, Baer. They are lucky to have a doctor that makes emergency night calls."

"Well, sir, the problem that's bothering me is not medical, it's really philosophical. After ten days, I tried sending Mrs. Stone home, but she was hopelessly confused and totally incontinent. She now needed an indwelling catheter [a rubber tube left permanently in the bladder], and enemas three times a week. Her obesity and total helplessness created too much of a nursing problem for Miss Stone and her part-time nurse. Full-time nursing at her home was too expensive, and so I had to put your old patient, Mrs. Stone, in a nursing home.

"Her mind is now entirely gone. I am sure the episode of heart failure produced additional brain damage and destroyed what little thinking capacity she still had.

"But her heart is back to normal rhythm, she is well compensated, and it seems to me she may exist in her present state of limbo for a year or two, for all I can see to the contrary.

"My problem is that I feel in part responsible for this predicament. It is depressing when I think it could last two more years. Her daughter goes to see her three times a week and is more distressed after each visit. I attempted to help, but I feel I have done more harm than good by my expert care.

"Old Mrs. Stone does not know where she is, but she knows she's not home and she is wretched most of the time. Her only question when I see her is, 'When can I go home?' I usually lie and say, 'Early next week,' hoping by next week she will have forgotten what I said.

"I guess my question is this, Dr. C., If you had made the house call, how would you have handled it?"

"Well, Baer, one of my thoughtful patients once asked me in considering this very type of problem, *'Do doctors know the real enemy?'* Sometimes I wonder if we do. It has been said that the retrospectoscope is the greatest medical instrument ever invented. Viewing this patient through its all-seeing lens, it seems you certainly did not improve her condition. As a matter of fact, you did indeed make it much worse. Without your treatment she would have died in a matter of minutes. That's what's bothering you, isn't it?"

"Yes, sir."

"Well, you said your problem was philosophical and I agree,

so let's look at it philosophically.

"In essence, you improved her heart function but not her human situation! Your treatment was not heroic, just good, standard, aggressive, medical management of her acute heart failure. Yet now you are sorry. The patient is miserable and depressed and her daughter is unhappy, not with you but with the outcome.

"Perhaps, Baer, you did battle with the wrong enemy. Her major disease was, and still is, her senile organic brain syndrome, which, we tend to forget, is less curable than metastatic cancer, and as inexorably progressive.

"As I understand it, your real question to me is how should you act the next time under similar circumstances. You can't just stand by and watch her die, can you?"

"That's right, sir."

"My first recommendation is that you try gradually to sound out your elderly patients, not at their first office visit, but after you have cared for them a year or so. At an appropriate time, raise the issue of a possible sudden, life-threatening emergency. Ask frankly how vigorous they want your life-preserving techniques to be. I have asked many of my patients this question. Almost all patients of mine in their seventies and eighties have said, 'Let me die quickly,' or, 'Let the good Lord take me.' After such a discussion with a patient I always make a handwritten note in the chart indicating the tenor of what was said.

"In a senile or semi-senile patient you must ask yourself and the patient's family this question long before the emergency arises. But there will still be times when you will have to judge for yourself. The patient may be unable to tell what is wished, and there may be no family in attendance.

"I have used the statement of my old friend, W. T. Longcope of Johns Hopkins as my guide. He said to me once in speaking of situations similar to Mrs. Stone's, 'Why ward off death if in the attempt we kill living?'[13]

"So to answer briefly how would I have treated Mrs. Stone, I would have acted more positively in a negative fashion. I would have given her a very small dose of aminophylline to help ease her breathing and a larger dose of morphine to help her rest and relieve her anxiety, I would have had her taken slowly to the hospital by ambulance, giving her small doses of oxygen en route so that her daughter could see she was being treated, not just left to die. I would have ordered private nurses so that there was always a human being in her room. If I gave her any additional digitalis or diuretics, I would have used very small doses—again enough for the daughter to see that her mother was being treated, but as the injections would have been too small to be very effective I believe that none of these actions of mine would have changed the fundamental problem of her heart failure.

"If she was still living by the next morning and had not died quietly, I would have had a consultant see her with me. If he agreed that under all the circumstances, nothing more should be done than what I had already ordered—to wit, sufficient morphine to relieve her shortness of breath, cough, apprehension, and to ensure sleep—then I would have asked the daughter to approve our joint recommendation. In addition, I would have continued the oxygen—more for the daughter than for the patient—and *nothing else!* I am sure Mrs. Stone, without full doses of digitalis and Mercuhydrin and aminophylline, would have died quietly in a week or less."

"That's easier to do, Dr. C., when you are Chief of the Department of Medicine and have a national reputation than when you are only thirty-two and are just starting out in practice."

"True, Baer, but that's why in a similar situation I suggest, while you are young, seek older doctors for consultation, and, if need be, two consultants. In my forty years in practice, liberal use of consultation has always been beneficial to my patients and their families, and to me. I have never had anyone complain because of my requesting a consultation."

In brief, that is the story of the first emergency patient of mine, who ended her life in a nursing home because of the treatment I administered.

Now, three decades later, when a similar problem arises, if there is any doubt as to whether to treat or not to treat an elderly, semi-senile patient vigorously, I lean toward mild measures. When there is any question in my own mind, I call a consultant. When I was young, I called older physicians in consultation. Now that I am the oldest member of the hospital staff, I call younger men.

I do not believe that in the past ten years any patient of mine has ended his or her life in a so-called convalescent hospital because of my aggressive medical measures. My older patients are nearly unanimous in telling me that "the real enemy" they most fear is senility, or total invalidism and confinement in a nursing home, *not* a sudden death or a short final illness.

I have just described how thirty years ago our relatively simple medicines quickly reversed the heart failure of an elderly woman patient of mine and prolonged for many months what became a meaningless existence. Just thirty years earlier than this, nothing could have been done. Today, thirty years later, you and I are faced with medical and technical measures one hundred times as effective for good or *for ill* as those I used for Mrs. Stone.

Recently it was my turn to read cardiograms for one of the finest hospitals on the West Coast staffed by an exceptionally able, dedicated, hardworking group of doctors, nurses, and technicians. Let me tell you about Mr. Hughes, a seventy-five-year-old man whose cardiogram I read. This is not an unusual case. It is duplicated more than a thousand times daily in this country.

Two months ago Mr. Hughes sustained a severe totally incapacitating heart attack. Due to heroic and expert hospital treatment he survived and eventually went home albeit a complete cardiac cripple. He had to rest in his hospital type of bed twenty-two hours out of each day, permanently! He was not senile, but he would never again regain strength or stamina because of the extensive damage to his heart.

At 2 A.M. yesterday morning, eight weeks after his first heart attack, he had another attack at home characterized by chest pain, shortness of breath, and total collapse.

His wife called their heart specialist. He summoned the special emergency ambulance staffed with paramedics. They gave him external cardiac massage and mouth-to-mouth breathing while rushing him to the emergency room.

In the emergency room his trachea (windpipe) was intubated, intravenous drugs were administered, and electrical countershock restored his heart to spontaneous beating (although feeble, rapid, and chaotic).

He was transferred to the intensive care unit, where four more times his heart ceased effective beating and four more times he was stimulated by drugs and shocked by an electrical current back to "life."

The doctors knew that his brain could have suffered severe damage. His wife was so informed, *but no one called a halt!*

I saw him at 9 P.M. last evening, nineteen hours after his admission to intensive care. He was partially paralyzed and could not understand the simplest command, such as "Make a fist." He is certain to be transferred to a nursing home if he is unfortunate enough to survive the next two weeks in the hospital.

This case is really typical of what is being done routinely to thousands of older patients in this country, with the best of intentions—with occasional brilliant success but far too often with the worst possible results.

There was no guilt in the scenario I have just described. The patient was a passive victim of science. His wife did her duty; the cardiologist did his; the paramedics in the ambulance did theirs; the emergency room doctors and nurses and the intensive care personnel did theirs. Why did it end so disastrously?

Because *the patient* had not considered long in advance the possibility of a heart attack and the pros and cons of aggressive treatment at his age and in his situation. He had made no decisions, given no orders—therefore, the doctors treated him heroically.

You assume responsibility for your life. If you would welcome a natural sudden death or a brief final illness, *you have to assume responsibility for the way you die.* If you don't, "the system" will take charge, and you may suffer consequences similar to those in the case of Mr. Hughes.

It is common practice today, even in people sixty-five, seventy, and seventy-five, to shock back into action a heart that may have ceased effective beating six times in one hour (with an unpredictable amount of consequent brain damage).

If that is what you want—fine, it will be done! If that is not what you want, then say so, LOUD and CLEAR.

# Chapter 6

## Treatment May Be Worse than Disease

> There was a woman "who had suffered much under many physicians . . . and was no better but rather grew worse."
>
> Mark 5:26

Patients over sixty-five whose chief problem is medical rather than surgical frequently discover that the treatment of their ailment is worse than the disease.

An incident occurred one Sunday morning that forcefully reminded me of this ancient doctrine, which is truer today than when first enunciated by Juvenal two thousand years ago.

I had been invited to speak to a church congregation on "The Therapeutic Value of Charity."

At the end of my presentation, after the usual question-and-answer period, a handsome, well-dressed woman in her early fifties approached me. I seemed to recall her face and when she spoke I was sure I had met her previously. I have a long memory for attractive women!

"Dr. Baer, I am Susan Winslow. Thirty years ago in San Francisco I was a student nurse and you taught our class on materia medica.

"Since then I have heard you speak several times and I just

wanted you to know that I agree with much of what you have to say in criticism of too much science and too little humanity in the medical treatment of some hospitalized patients. I was a coronary care unit nurse for eight years and I have just resigned. I couldn't take it anymore."

After thanking the program chairman for inviting me to speak, I asked my former student to join me at my favorite fresh doughnut shop for further conversation.

Susan, as I said, was attractive. She was warm, intelligent, articulate, and anxious to talk about the experiences she had had on the coronary care unit which had led to her resignation and return to private duty nursing. It is difficult to obtain a sampling of opinion regarding some of the controversial and emotionally charged questions that arise in connection with modern coronary care units. The largest nursing journal in this country would not print a letter of mine in which I requested answers to a questionnaire concerning resuscitation and the mechanized prolongation of biological existence. In personal interviews I have always found nurses willing to be utterly frank in expressing illuminating feelings and value judgments.

## THE CORONARY CARE UNIT

The CCU nurses are some of the finest in any hospital and they receive considerable extra salary for their work. Susan's resignation therefore had an element of financial sacrifice, which is some indication of how strongly she felt about the matter.

A coronary care unit is designed to monitor electrically every beat of a patient's heart twenty-four hours a day as long as the patient is on the unit. The electrocardiogram of each patient is visible at all times (by telemetry) to the coronary care unit personnel sitting at the central nursing station. Every heartbeat of every patient on the unit is recorded.

If a cardiac arrest or a life-threatening abnormal rate or

rhythm develops, there is a warning system to alert the nurses to respond immediately by following "standing CCU emergency orders."

When a patient is first admitted to the unit, a continuous intravenous drip is started. Immediately upon the detection of an abnormal rate or rhythm, appropriate drugs are administered into the intravenous tube to try to prevent more serious abnormalities. In the case of a cardiac arrest mouth-to-mouth resuscitation, external cardiac massage, or electroshock cardioversion are instituted. Much of this is now started by the coronary care unit nurses. In addition, the telephone operators are alerted and page all doctors in the hospital to come immediately to assist. They may institute endotracheal intubation (the placing of a tube beyond the vocal cords into the windpipe), begin mechanical respiratory assistance or artificial heart-pacing with an electronic pacemaker. A battery of blood tests and further intravenous medications will continue for half an hour minimum and up to two hours if no one orders a halt.

When the system works well, and the patient is in the thirties, forties, or fifties, a life may be saved and the patient may leave the hospital in good health and with adequate, if not complete, strength and stamina. These cases alone well justify the enormous expense of time and money involved in building, supplying, and staffing the thousands of coronary care units now operating in America.

On the other hand, many an older patient or chronically ill patient is admitted to the CCU and the results are undesirable. After ten years of growing utilization, many physicians and even some cardiologists are questioning whether for the older patient the drawbacks of the CCU may not outweigh its advantages.

A recently published article entitled "Evaluating Medical Technology," by Osler L. Peterson, M.D., F.A.C.P., of the Department of Preventive and Social Medicine, Harvard Medical School, states:

Some cardiologists, presumably a minority, are skeptical about coronary care unit effectiveness. *Their* skepticism is well based.[14]

If you are over seventy-five, or have had a previous heart attack, or have some other major medical problem, I believe you should carefully consider a non coronary care unit bed if you suffer a coronary occlusion!

If you do not fear the possibility of sudden death and in fact prefer this mode of dying to possibly having to exist, but not live, after heroic treatment on the CCU, discuss this with your doctor now while you are able and both of you have the time.

If you wait for the attack, there will be no time for either of you to reflect.

It will all be action and you will probably be too sick to partake in any important decisions. Others will have to make them for you—perhaps to your sorrow.

When we reached the doughnut shop, Susan and I sat down in a vacant booth. I sipped some coffee and said, "Tell me why you resigned."

"We had two patients last month, Dr. Baer, on the coronary care unit at the same time. For six months I have discussed with my husband the possibility of resigning. These two patients were the final straw that brought me to tender my resignation."

## THE CASE OF DR. G.

"Dr. G. was one of the best psychiatrists on our staff. He was seventy-one years old. His heart attack occurred in his office. A manic patient threatened him with a loaded gun for half an hour before his secretary, realizing from the man's loud voice that something serious was amiss, called the police. They overpowered the patient, but just as they were leaving, the doctor began to have crushing chest pain radiating to his jaw. He knew, of course, what had happened and asked the police to call an ambulance and told his secretary to call his wife.

"He was admitted to our coronary care unit fifteen minutes after the onset of his attack. The pain increased during the next four hours and his electrocardiogram and blood tests confirmed the diagnosis of a very serious myocardial infarction.

"Not unexpectedly, he developed ventricular fibrillation [a fatal complication] ten hours after admission, with cardiac arrest and profound shock. His blood pressure was not obtainable. We defibrillated [electric shock to the heart] him seven times and continued external cardiac massage for over an hour. We had three alternating teams. We gave him mouth-to-mouth respiration for twenty minutes. When spontaneous respiration did not occur we used a hand-operated bag to inflate his lungs for two hours.

"Following successful restoration of spontaneous heart-beating [a so-called viable rhythm], we called an anesthesiologist to intubate him [place a tube into the windpipe]. He was attached to an intermittent positive pressure breathing machine for the first forty-eight hours. Then, and because we were having trouble with his endotracheal tube, the surgeons were asked to perform a tracheostomy [a surgical hole made through the neck into the windpipe]. He was continued on the automatic respirator while every drug I had ever seen used or heard of was employed intravenously to maintain his blood pressure, which hovered around the shock area. His pulse during this time was nearly imperceptible.

"The third day he developed convulsions lasting two hours which required yet other intravenous medication to stop.

"The fourth day the X-rays showed pneumonia and he was placed on antibiotics. Really, it seemed as though every twenty minutes we were injecting one drug or another into his intravenous tubing.

"I know that his wife, who was a former high school biology teacher, asked the doctors on three different occasions during the first week if her husband's brain would be damaged if he survived the attack. She was told that as his eyes would open, his pupils responded, and he could move a leg or an arm if it were pricked with a pin that there was hope. She asked why then he could not breathe by himself. Did not that mean severe damage to the respiratory center? 'Yes,' said his doctors, but no one could or would turn off the respiratory assistance machine so long as there was any evidence of brain activity. 'We are not here to play God,' was the laconic reply of his attending cardiologist.

"It seems that anyone can flip on the switch of that terrible machine but only God can turn it off! It's really frightful making rounds on a service where three of those machines are going all the time, 'pst-chew, pst-chew, pst-chew,' day and night.

"On the tenth day he began to respond to simple commands such as 'Squeeze my fingers, Stick out your tongue, Open your eyes.' I hated going into his room and looking at his eyes. He really had had a penetrating glance; now his eyes just looked without seeing. They would kind of 'track' without understanding what they saw, like a six-week-old infant.

"He required mechanical assistance for breathing for a total of two weeks. By the end of a month his mind had made only a slow and very limited recovery. Therefore, he was transferred to the 'rehabilitation service.' There he made little progress, and six weeks later was sent to a nursing home. He was so confused in his thinking that he required twenty-four hour-a-day supervision which was impossible at home.

"Two months later he developed shortness of breath and wheezing and was transferred back to the hospital, where X-rays showed the trachea was scarred from the intubation tube [always a possibility, not malpractice]. It had become so narrow due to the scarring that air would not pass, hence the wheeze. He was not on our coronary care unit at that time, but I went by his room each day to see him. I couldn't help him but I knew my visits helped his wife.

"He was brought back to the hospital once every three weeks for a dilation of his windpipe in an attempt to widen it. These were painful and exhausting procedures which left him prostrate.

"Finally, six months later he had a permanent tracheostomy [a permanent hole in the windpipe], so that he could breathe. He shuts this off with his finger when he tries to talk.

"He is still in the nursing home, as his brain is so damaged it would be too hazardous to leave him at home. He is a smoker and could easily set the house afire, having less judgment about matches than a four-year-old.

"His wife has gone back to teaching to help pay for his more than one-thousand-a-month nursing home bill. I am sure he will live several more years as he is unless he has another heart attack soon."

## A WORD ABOUT PACEMAKERS

Susan's second case dealt with a pacemaker. These are a boon to tens of thousands of patients in their forties, fifties, sixties, and even seventies, who are otherwise strong and vigorous. When such patients develop partial or total heart block with long pauses, or an extremely low pulse rate (thirty to forty beats per minute), or unpredictable changes in heart rate (from very slow to very fast), the pacemaker takes over.

But the results of a pacemaker implant in patients in their eighties and nineties is another matter. It must be said that many of these patients, even at this age, have good results. But many others have ended with a pacemaker implacably triggering seventy beats a minute in the previously crippled heart while the brain that it nourishes deteriorates from the complications of age.

A pacemaker can be a boon, but it can, unless the mind is

alert, be a great disaster. Sometimes it is better in your old age to submit to the restrictions imposed by heart block, live quietly at home, and eventually die a natural death from heart failure than to be fitted with a pacemaker that no one can stop until it wears out months or years after you have become senile.

## THE CASE OF DR. D.

Susan resumed, "The second patient that keeps haunting me was also a professional man. He was emeritus professor of physics at our most distinguished Bay Area university. He was the former head of the department, internationally famous. His doctor told me one day that Professor D. was the most brilliant man he had every known.

"A friend of my husband's was a former student of Professor D.'s and a member of his department for many years. He told us the personal story behind the purely medical history dictated by his doctor for the hospital record.

"Professor D. had remained active through his eightieth year. By 1974, when he was eighty-five years old, he began to suffer the complication of the diabetes he had had for many years. He lost most of his sight because of diabetic deterioration of the retina, and simultaneously his hearing diminished, so that in spite of hearing aids he could not understand even when someone spoke directly into his ear. He could no longer read even the large print *Reader's Digest,* which my husband's friend used to bring to him. Soon he had to stop going for walks, which had been his lifetime exercise, and he retired into his study withdrawn from friends, life, and even his wife.

"By this time they were both eighty-six. She could not visit him in his study, because severe arthritis of her knees made the stair climb to his quarters impossible.

"In early 1976, Professor D. developed total heart block. His pulse dropped to 32 beats a minute, he took to his bed and would not even sit up in a chair for meals. His doctor, a good physician, recommended a pacemaker. His wife refused to give permission, but finally assented when much medical pressure was brought to bear. She really knew better than the doctors. She had been married to him for more than sixty years, but her advanced age and a previous stroke had enfeebled her and left her without sufficient energy or strength to argue with the doctors and to forbid the pacemaker implantation. They had no children.

"He was taken by ambulance to our hospital and admitted to my ward for cardiac monitoring of his heart block.

"After three days' observation, a pacemaker was implanted. The operation was successful but the patient's condition was unchanged except that his pulse rate was now 70 instead of 32.

"Late last year his wife died of a second stroke, so that he had to be moved to a nursing home.

"Six weeks ago I was visiting my aunt in this nursing home. She was recovering from a recently fractured hip. The nurse told me Professor D. was there, and I went to his room to see him. There he was—diapered, turned from side to side on a water bed mattress to prevent bedsores. I took his pulse—it was 70, still being triggered by his damn pacemaker! I could not get him out of my mind. I submitted my two weeks' notice to our Chief of Nursing the next day!"

## CORONARY CARE FOR OLDER PATIENTS

These two case histories are not at all unusual. They illustrate that for many older patients, the treatment that one receives in the coronary care unit can in spite of the best intentions be worse than the disease.

I have carefully considered for myself the Yin and the Yang sides of being cared for in a coronary care unit should I have a coronary occlusion. When I pass the age of seventy, I will choose a private room, or if I am not too sick, I will remain at home. At my present age of sixty-four I would go to the CCU with the strict "patients orders" you will find discussed in detail in Chapters 11 and 12.

Other doctors see it a little differently. A brilliant cardiologist age fifty-five whom I know said to me that he would go to the coronary care unit for only seventy-two hours, chiefly for the prevention or correction of serious abnormal heart rhythms. The younger men generally want the "full treatment." The overwhelming majority of the older doctors would place strict limits on the routine resuscitation attempts which are a built-in feature of all coronary care units.

My patients in their early sixties who are strong and vigorous and have never known a sick day in their lives usually feel that the promise of positive Yang results of treatment in a coronary care unit sufficiently outweigh the less well known negative Yin risks of such treatment.

The vast majority of my older patients, those in their eighties and nineties, choose not to be admitted to the coronary care unit. Those in their seventies who have already experienced serious medical problems also choose to decline such care. These patients agree with me that if you survive a coronary occlusion naturally and make a good recovery with only minor supportive measures—which 80 percent of all such patients do —that's good enough. Every one of them hopes to have his or her heart cease before senility overtakes the mind.

As Dr. Charles D. Aring, of the College of Medicine of the University of Cincinnati, has said, "Death can be natural if we will make it so."[15]

# Chapter 7

## How Much Is Enough?

> Medicine is practiced defensively, with every known technique used. Thus, the hospital administrator or a doctor can say that he did everything possible to save the patient.
>
> Roland Stevens, M.D., *People's Weekly Magazine,* March 17, 1976

### THE EMERGENCY ROOM

If you are suddenly stricken with illness or involved in an accident, you will find yourself in another of those marvels of modern medicine—the emergency room.

The emergency room staff of doctors, nurses, and technicians in any well-run modern hospital is trained and equipped to render you the most expert emergency care available. It is prompt, skillful, efficient, and available twenty-four hours a day, seven days a week.

If your situation is serious, it is likely that you will arrive at the emergency room by ambulance, without your own doctor having been notified in advance. He will not be able to meet you there or telephone instructions ahead of his arrival. And if you are unable, due to your illness, to communicate your own thoughts to the doctor on duty, then matters are taken totally out of your hands.

Under these circumstances you have no control over what treatment you receive, how prolonged it will be, or how aggressive.

The doctors and nurses in the emergency room have no way of discovering your desires, and no time to try to do so. They are expertly trained and equipped to preserve the vital functioning of your heart and lungs. This they will do, if possible—speedily, aggressively, and skillfully, with every modern technical, medical, and surgical means available. There is no one to say "Don't!" There is no one to say "Stop!" All the pressure is TO DO!

In the emergency room, decisions must be instantaneous and actions must be carried out *immediately.* There is no time for reflection!

This may all turn out well. But if you are in your later years, it may turn out disastrously for you! It could be the direct cause of your spending months or years totally dependent and demented in an extended care facility.

Twenty-five years ago, when an elderly person was suddenly taken seriously ill at home, the doctor was called to the house. The doctor would come, ascertain that the illness would probably result in death in a matter of hours or a day or so, give the patient morphine to ease the pain and anxiety, call a nurse to come in and give care at home, and continue the morphine as needed. Soon death from natural causes would quietly occur in the person's own bed.

With the advent of the modern emergency room, the radio-dispatched paramedical-staffed and equipment-jammed ambulance, and Medicare to pick up the tab, there is a different scenario. The patient, the family, a friend, a neighbor, or the doctor, orders an ambulance. The patient is picked up and brought immediately to the emergency room, where the full impact of modern science goes into action. Too often the result merely prolongs biological existence and all too often ensures a process of dying that may take weeks, months, or even years.

I am determined not to let this happen to me! If you agree with my point of view, it need not happen to you.

Cardiopulmonary resuscitation (CPR) is a relatively new technique. In the past ten years it has become *mandatory* for every doctor to learn and practice it so that he can pass a yearly qualifying test on a dummy model. At present, cardiopulmonary resuscitation receives widespread medical and public support and press coverage. But as with every newly invented technique from the wheel to atomic energy, it takes much longer to discover the Yin than the Yang in the new discovery.

There is no question that for a young person who suffers cardiopulmonary arrest in a swimming pool accident and who has been observed immediately and can be promptly rescued, cardiopulmonary resuscitation can be lifesaving and usually health-restoring. A young person can withstand an oxygen deficiency to the brain far better and far longer than someone over sixty-five. But even so, every summer many young Americans are resuscitated who later are found to have minimal, moderate, and sometimes severe brain damage. Nevertheless, cardiopulmonary resuscitation is frequently of dramatic value for a young person in the thirties, forties, or fifties whose cardiac arrest is instantly observed and promptly and expertly treated, all within four minutes maximum. Scores of such younger cardiac patients are successfully resuscitated and eventually discharged in good, if not perfect, health every week in this country.

But for the person over sixty-five who suffers a sudden cardiopulmonary arrest at home or at work, it is apt to be a far different story. I recently polled sixty physicians as to their desire if they sustained an *unobserved* cardiac arrest (i.e., one not instantly noted). Every doctor in his thirties wanted a full half hour's attempt to resuscitate. Every doctor over sixty wanted no attempt. The latter did not want to have the heart and respiration restarted only to exist for months or years with an incurably damaged brain. Far better to be dead than demented.

Resuscitation is routine in every American hospital for every patient unless the doctor has left written orders to the contrary. How this works out in the case of older patients, and the dilemmas that face patient and doctor alike, is illustrated in what follows.

## SPECIAL MEETING OF DOCTORS

A special doctors meeting has been called for 7:30 A.M. The hospital is being sued for $1,500,000. A woman patient of forty developed cardiac arrest in the operating room. She was resuscitated, but her brain was permanently damaged. Therefore, she is no longer able to function as a wife, a mother, and a housekeeper. Her husband has filed suit.

The hospital administration has asked each department to review all cases of attempted cardiopulmonary resuscitation in patients on their service from ages two to ninety, and to suggest to the executive committee guidelines for the future. The purpose is not to prevent cardiopulmonary arrest, which is impossible, but to prevent if possible further lawsuits against the hospital.

At precisely 7:30 A.M., Dr. H., chairman of the medical department, called the meeting to order. He is fifty-two, an exceptionally well liked, well trained, hardworking, and highly regarded internist, with a broad view on the problems of medicine, modern hospitals, and his patients.

"Let me have your attention, please," said Dr. H. "We have much to do this morning. You have been told that this special meeting will last for an hour and a half. It will end promptly at 9 A.M. Many of you have already asked to speak. I shall limit all remarks to five minutes.

"As you know, we have been asked to suggest guidelines for

the emergency room panel of physicians in the matter of instituting and carrying out attempted cardiopulmonary resuscitation.

"Each of us has his own ideas, and we know that each case has its own special problems, but nevertheless we must try to formulate a few suggestions, not rules, for the doctor first attending the cardiopulmonary arrest patient in the emergency room.

"I will give you briefly two case histories taken from the past month's emergency room log and chosen by our ad hoc committee as a basis for discussion. No criticism of the doctors involved is implied.

"The ad hoc committee believes you will perhaps find fault with one doctor for acting too vigorously and with the other doctor for stopping attempted cardiopulmonary resuscitation too soon. At least, these two histories should generate some useful discussion which I shall try to keep from being too heated."[16]

### THE FIRST CASE

The patient is a seventy-six-year-old widow. One evening at 9:55, she was found collapsed in her bathroom by the boarder who lived in her home. He was awakened by curious noises in the house. What he heard was the widow falling to the bathroom floor and her subsequent stertorous breathing.

The boarder called the Fire Department. They came and gave the comatose patient oxygen and called the ambulance, which got her to our emergency room at 10:14 P.M. The emergency room doctor on duty noted that just as the electrocardiographic monitor was being hooked up, the patient's respiration suddenly ceased and she became cyanotic (blue). On examination, he noted faint heart sound but could not feel her pulse nor obtain her blood pressure. She remained in a deep coma.

He immediately began mouth-to-mouth artificial respiration, and later had a nurse continue with a hand-operated bag ventilator. The patient's color improved somewhat.

The electrocardiographic monitor showed only a rapid heart rate and no evidence of a coronary occlusion ("heart attack" with damage to heart muscle).

On the patient's admission to the emergency room, a continuous intravenous drip had been started by the emergency room nurse. Every standard scientifically correct drug in the appropriate concentration was added to the solution, and dripping was at the prescribed rate. Every two or three minutes the doctor ordered the nurse to add further medication to the intravenous. All is precisely noted on the record.

Soon a stronger heartbeat was audible and the patient's pulse could be felt. Her blood pressure was obtainable fifteen minutes after she arrived in the emergency room, but she remained in a deep coma and did not respond to painful stimuli. Her pupils reacted, but sluggishly. She did not open her eyes spontaneously (a sign of deep coma).

Meanwhile, the police searched her bathroom and found there an old prescription. Unfortunately the doctor whose name was on it had retired from practice two years previously.

Her daughter's telephone number in New York City was in her address book, which was found by the police.

At 10:30 P.M., about one half hour after the patient's collapse had been heard by her boarder, a neurologist who had been called in consultation concurred with the tentative diagnosis of a subarachnoid hemorrhage (blood between the skull and the brain) after performing a lumbar puncture and finding blood cells in the spinal fluid.

Forty-five minutes after the patient had been admitted to the emergency room, her daughter was reached by telephone and told of her mother's desperate situation. She said: "Do whatever is indicated. I will fly out in the morning."

As the patient's respirations were becoming labored, an intermittent positive pressure breathing machine was substituted for the hand-operated bag ventilator. From now on, the mechanical respiratory assistance machine kept her breathing.

In spite of all efforts her coma deepened. The pupils no longer responded to light and remained dilated. At 11:30 P.M., after neurosurgical consultation with an extremely capable young neurosurgeon, it was decided to take X-rays of the blood vessels to her brain, and a radiopaque dye was injected into a neck artery. The angiogram (X-ray of the brain's arteries) confirmed the diagnosis of a subarachnoid hemorrhage due to the rupture of a weak spot in one of the blood vessels of the brain.

The neurosurgeon recommended craniotomy (opening of the skull), with an attempt to clamp the bleeding artery. This was begun at 1:30 A.M. and was completed by 4:30 A.M.

The surgery was successful, but the patient remained comatose.

She was transferred to the intensive care unit and for ten days received vigorous supportive measures, including continuous intravenous drip and continuous mechanical respiratory assistance and daily monitoring of her blood chemistry.

By the end of this time, her coma lightened slightly. She moved when she felt pain. Her pupils responded normally and her eyes opened. A permanent tracheostomy had been performed, as the intubation tube no longer functioned well.

On the fourth day in the intensive care unit, she had developed a very rapid, abnormal, potentially fatal heart rhythm. This persisted for three hours and did not respond to the usual intravenous drugs.

Finally, electrical shock was used, and after the third attempt a normal heartbeat was restored.

After ten days she was transferred to a regular hospital room, but further improvement was slow and limited.

She could respond to simple questions with monosyllables

but she could not express herself. She could not feed herself and was finally discharged to a nursing home four weeks after having been admitted to the emergency room.

It was the opinion of two members of the ad hoc committee, after reviewing this case and considering the woman's age and the very severe brain damage indicated by her original examination and deep coma, that the neurosurgery and the intensive care that followed were ill-advised and the direct cause of the patent's invalidism and nursing home confinement. The minority opinion was that the doctors in charge did what conformed to the daughter's instruction to do what was "indicated."

Dr. H. paused for a minute and said: "Please withhold all comments until I have given you the second case history. Because of the particularly controversial nature of this case, I shall read directly from the hospital record, with no comments of mine."

## THE SECOND CASE

The first page was the emergency room admission sheet. It stated that the patient was a fifty-nine-year-old male, brought to the emergency room by ambulance and clocked in at *13:06.* The ambulance driver's report stated that a telephone call had come from the public library at *13:01,* reporting that a man in a wheelchair had collapsed on the sidewalk in front of the library.

When they arrived, the patient was still breathing but they could not obtain a pulse or blood pressure. They thumped his chest once, with no response, and started external cardiac massage. En route to the hospital, his breathing stopped and they instituted mouth-to-mouth respiration. It was obvious to them that he had fallen out of his wheelchair which was overturned onto the sidewalk. The ambulance paramedics continued mouth-to-mouth resuscitation and external cardiac massage until they were relieved by the emergency room personnel.

The patient's identification card in his wallet revealed his home telephone number and that his wife was next of kin. She was called but there was no answer. The emergency card in his wallet stated that Dr. A. was his physician. Dr. A. was reached by telephone at his home and stated that he would be at the emergency room in five minutes. Meanwhile, the emergency room personnel remained in charge, as no one can give orders who is not on the scene.

The emergency room nurses' report ended with the notation: "Intravenous [listing four different drugs] started at *13:08*. EKG monitor revealed ventricular fibrillation." [This is a fatal, abnormal rhythm unless treated successfully in four minutes or less.]

Dr. H. read next from the emergency room doctor's report. It stated that the patient was cold, clammy, and cyanotic [blue]. His pupils were dilated; pulse and blood pressure were not obtainable. The doctor confirmed the EKG diagnosis of ventricular fibrillation and ordered the administration of 400 watts direct current countershock, which caused cessation of the ventricular fibrillation. This was followed by a few abnormal heartbeats. A hand-operated bag ventilator was substituted for mouth-to-mouth respiration; a continuous intravenous drip containing the newest drugs recommended by the coronary care committee was continued without restoring normal heart action, which again reverted to ventricular fibrillation.

At *13:10*, a second 400-watt countershock produced regular but very rapid, weak heartbeat. At *13:13*, ventricular fibrillation recurred, the patient was pulseless. External cardiac massage was again started.

At *13:15*, fourteen minutes after the original ambulance call, the patient's own doctor arrived. Two minutes later, after assessing the situation, he assumed responsibility and ordered all attempts at resuscitation discontinued.

Dr. H. then said, "I will finish this presentation by reading the patient's family doctor's note on the chart:

" 'This fifty-nine-year-old man and his wife have been patients of mine for over twenty years.'

" 'He has had slowly progressing multiple sclerosis since age thirty-one. Because of this he has been unable to work for the past two decades that I have cared for him. He has been unable to walk for ten years. His wife works full time, and once a week, on Saturdays, takes him in a wheelchair two blocks to the small park in front of the city library, where she leaves him while she shops. One of the young librarians steps outside every thirty minutes or so to be sure he is all right.

" 'In the past four years he has gotten so heavy and helpless that on those many occasions when he has fallen to the floor, his wife has required the aid of her neighbors, lately with increasing frequency, to help get him back into his wheelchair or into his bed. Furthermore, in the past six months his toilet needs have become so demanding and so physically difficult that his wife has spoken to me on three different occasions about her need to finally place him in a nursing home. She has not raised this issue with her husband, but had planned to have me tell him of the necessity of this transfer after his sixtieth birthday next month.

" 'It was therefore my judgment, as the family doctor, that the standard half-hour, all-out attempt to resuscitate this man would not be correct. As his wife was shopping and could not be reached, I took the full responsibility of stopping all CPR, I pronounced him dead at *13:17,* eleven minutes after he had been clocked into the emergency room.' "

## THE DOCTORS DISCUSS THE CASES

Dr. H. opened the meeting for discussion. He decided to recognize those who wanted to speak in turn alphabetically.

That made me the first to comment.

I said:

"I wish vigorously to concur with the decision to stop cardiopulmonary resuscitation in the second case. It seems to me that instead of the large printed sign in the emergency room which states, 'Your hospital bill does not include your doctor's bill,' we should have a larger one reading, 'When there is any doubt whatsoever that the action you are about to undertake is for the welfare of the patient, abstain' [Zoroaster]."

Dr. Bird was next.

"If Dr. Baer had been taken to court as I was and sued by the litigious son of a long-retired accountant—who had already had two strokes—for not trying to resuscitate him, he might feel differently.

"I won my suit, but I was in court for ten days, cross-examined for two hours in the witness chair, and spent more than two hundred hours helping my attorney prepare my defense!

"Now I try to resuscitate every one of my patients for no less than thirty minutes."

Dr. Davidoff was next.

"I would like to know whose welfare we are here to consider. The patient's, the doctors', the hospital, or the insurance company? I was under the impression the patient's welfare was the only reason for building and equipping a hospital in the first place. At least, that's what Maimonides, the greatest Jewish physician who ever lived, would have said eight hundred years ago in his *Guide for the Perplexed.*"

Dr. Kelley commented.

"Well, I don't know about Maimonides, but I do know what Pope Pius XII said. He stated the doctor need not use extraordinary means to keep life going, and that's what I think was done in the first case you presented."

Dr. Kim, a member of the emergency room panel.

"Well, gentlemen, I can't quote any sage advice from Lao-tse or Mencius, but I wish to call your attention to the fact that those of us on the panel are working under incredible pressure with no time to consider philosophic matters. Nine tenths of the emergencies are upon us before any member of the family or the patient's doctor knows a thing about what's going on. The patient is usually comatose, stuporous, confused, or too sick to give us any guidance."

Mr. Manley, of the hospital administration.

"Gentlemen, the administration asked me to say that if the hospital is going to continue to help pay malpractice premiums for the emergency room panel, it must have a statement of policy from the medical staff and have this approved by the executive committee and the board of directors.

"I know that the administrator and the hospital's attorney feel that the most important item in defending ourselves against a suit is to have *all the details carefully noted in the record.*

"Before modern advanced techniques were available, a hospital was hardly ever sued. As recently as ten years ago a suit against this hospital was unknown. If the patient died, everyone had done his best; death was an expected complication of major surgery and serious illness. But that's not true today.

"Truly, our chief worry is still not the patient who dies in spite of your best efforts but the one who is resuscitated and lives on but as a total invalid."

Dr. Oppenheim, also on the emergency room panel.

"It's all well and good for the administration to want a detailed written report of each case. Our panel may see fifty patients in the twenty-four hours we are on duty. I have partaken in prolonged, difficult cardiopulmonary resuscitation attempts that have lasted two hours. It is very hard to include all the details of such an attempt even with a nurse assigned to do just that.

"Former President Truman is reported to have said, 'If you can't stand the heat, get out of the kitchen.' Well, I am young, very well trained, and amply endowed with energy. I know what I'm doing in an emergency. But the pressure for perfect results and perfect documentation is unreal. I have thought and even talked with my wife about resigning and joining the Navy Medical Corps, where I would have no suits, no malpractice premium to pay, and a forty-hour week!"

Dr. May, a cardiologist.

"I agree with Dr. Oppenheim. The emergency room is vastly different from the coronary care unit. We on the coronary care unit know our patients and their family. For the most part, we know their opinion. But I should just like to call your attention to the official policy of the American Heart Association. It is official, it is published. The AHA is a wealthy and highly regarded group. It promulgates its opinions widely. I think that those of you who don't know what the AHA recommends should inform yourselves, even though you may disagree. You can be certain that every malpractice attorney knows exactly what the American Heart Association has to say!

"Briefly, the American Heart Association policy states that if you do not know *positively and absolutely* that the patient's brain is permanently damaged beyond all hope, you must give him the benefit of the doubt and immediately institute vigorous and, if necessary, prolonged attempts at cardiopulmonary resuscitation.

"That means, in short, that any patient brought to the emergency room who previously would have been diagnosed as 'dead on arrival' (DOA); who has no history, no family, no personal physician on hand—as they usually do not—no matter if the patient is two or ninety-two, you damn well better start cardiopulmonary resuscitation the minute the body comes through the door.

"You may not agree, as I have said, but it is the official American Heart Association policy."

Dr. Pavlovsky, eighty years old, who practiced family medicine for fifty years.

"Gentlemen, it seems to me the wrong people are making policy. We have heard from emergency room specialists, heart specialists, administrators, and we still have not heard from respiratory disease specialists, gastroenterologists, neurologists, nephrologists, or oncologists!

"Why doesn't someone ask the *patients* what they want? The trouble is, the poor patient does not know what's in store for him when he's rushed from the ambulance through those automatic doors into a resuscitation room. I think all the experts—and I'm glad we have them—should make suggestions and act as consultants, but I think this hospital's policy regarding older patients should be made by those men who are in family practice or general internal medicine. They are the ones most apt to follow a patient along for many years and come to know what he really wants and what he really fears. But, of course, I know this won't happen!"

"Well, as a first step, Dr. Pavlovsky, will you serve on the committee to help draw up our recommendations?" asked Dr. H.

"Yes, sir."

Mrs. Eaton, head emergency room nurse for five years.

"Frankly, if the general public could be present at a few cardiopulmonary resuscitation attempts, I think there would be a different view than now prevails. It can be a brutal experience. The patient is usually very cyanotic; he is apt to be gray-haired. The odor of burnt flesh from the electrode paddles added to the odor of urine and fecal matter from incontinence or that of vomitus is not present when resuscitation is shown on the TV screen or in educational movies.

"And though I have seen occasional, brilliant, and unexpectedly good results in the young and middle-aged, most of the time in older patients where there has been a true cardiopulmonary arrest [cessation of both heartbeat and respiration], attempted resuscitation is not a rewarding experience. It is, instead, frustrating, unnerving, traumatic, and truly gruesome!

"I think I can sum up my feelings and that of most of my nurses when I tell you that the morning after Dr. Y. had ordered cardiopulmonary resuscitation stopped in the instance of the second patient you described, I was on duty and went up to him and thanked him for the courage and humanity he had shown in saying, 'STOP,' and pronouncing the patient dead. Not many younger men on the staff would have done that!"

Chaplain Ratcliffe, with long hospital affiliation.

"I think the problem that confronts you is one of the few that I have seen in which the Sermon on the Mount is not helpful.

"If you do unto your patients as you would be done by, you may be substituting your value judgment of life and living for theirs.

"Somehow, before the crisis is upon you and your patient, you have to have insight into an unknown person's mind in an unpredictable situation.

"That's asking a lot. It's apparent we need to educate the older members of our society to tell their doctor *while they are well* what they hope he *won't* do if they become suddenly desperately ill or are gravely injured.

"I agree with Robert Veatch,[17] who emphasizes time and

again that in the midst of the present biological revolution patients must now assume the imperative task of seeking for themselves a responsible role in the medical decisions affecting their own death or dying."

While the doctors cast unsigned votes on the two cases, Dr. H. made the following summary comments:

"It seems to me that one authority who has not been quoted this morning is an immortal physician whose dictum has stood for twenty-five hundred years.

"Hippocrates' teaching, translated from his Greek into Latin, said, *'Primum non nacera,'* 'In the *first* place do no harm.'

"I believe we sometimes lose sight of this when in our efforts to help a patient by resuscitation we inadvertently do great harm.

"I would like to suggest that the Department of Medicine go on record as advocating this rule as a chief guideline in any policy statement adopted by this hospital in regard to cardiopulmonary resuscitation in the emergency room."

How would you vote? Was the effort in the first case too prolonged? In the second, stopped too soon? What policies do you think the emergency room personnel should follow in attempting to resuscitate older patients?

The doctors thought the treatment in the first case too aggressive by a vote of 29 to 19; they felt it was too short in the second by a vote of 26 to 16.

# Chapter 8

## The Elusive Diagnosis

> Death is both a friend and an enemy. . . . We have a basic
> human right in certain circumstances to decide for our-
> selves when it is one more than the other.

> Rev. A. B. Downing, cited in
> *Euthanasia,* December 1977

### YOU ARE INVITED TO A CLINICAL
### PATHOLOGICAL CONFERENCE

A clinical pathological conference is the great tour de force
of a modern teaching hospital and medical school. It is akin to
the coda in a violin concerto. It gives the discussant a chance
to show off his diagnostic acumen, the breadth of his clinical
learning, and the depth of his anatomic, physiologic, and
pathologic understanding.

It is the classical "whodunit" in a medical setting!

A patient is chosen whose diagnosis has completely stumped
the interns, the residents, the radiologists, and the medical staff
attending the case. If the correct diagnosis is finally established
by surgery, or if the patient dies and the diagnosis is determined
by autopsy, "the case" may be used for a CPC.

If it is, then several months later, after all talk about the "interesting case" has ceased, a distinguished visitor is given the patient's history, the findings on examination, and the laboratory and X-ray data, and is asked to discuss the diagnosis in front of the whole faculty and student body at a clinical pathological conference.

Recently I was asked to be the visiting professor of medical ethics for one week at an Eastern university and discuss such a case. The materials given to me contained all the necessary clues, with perhaps a few red herrings thrown in.

Clinical pathological conferences are popular and well attended. They are excellent means of teaching the pitfalls of diagnosis as well as the proper method of "working up a case" —that is, what questions to ask the patient, what tests and X-rays to order, and in what sequence.

The most instructive of the clinical pathological conferences are printed in their entirety in the best medical journals.

If you are the patient, over sixty-five, and have a rare disease, or an unusual complication, or your diagnosis is obscure, you had better beware! In the attempt to "work your case up thoroughly," a new hazardous test or treatment which may inadvertently cause you to suffer a complication may be used. Or you may experience needless prolongation of a chronic illness when the doctors try "everything in the book," in the name of Science and Research, to treat an obscure or essentially incurable disease.

It is true that at teaching hospitals patients can receive the most advanced medical and surgical treatment in this country. But if you are over sixty-five, the most advanced treatment may not be the best for you. University hospital patients in their seventies and eighties are not all cured! Frequently they too are transferred to nursing homes, where their long-term course is followed by their family doctor but may soon be forgotten by the busy full-time teaching and research staff of the medical school.

This is a brief summary of the case I was asked to discuss at the CPC.

## CASE HISTORY

The patient was a sixty-three-year-old male admitted to the intensive care unit of the university hospital. The chief complaints were coughing up blood for one day, increasing shortness of breath, extreme fatigue, and weight loss for several months. A week before admission he was unable to dress himself without severe shortness of breath.

He was chronically ill, a severely and increasingly incapacitated man.

He had been a heavy cigarette smoker—up to two packs a day—since age eighteen. In addition, he had been exposed to much asbestos in his work at a firm that specialized in the destruction of old frame houses.

By the time he was fifty-seven, he was forced to retire because of severe bronchitis, emphysema, and asbestosis (a chronic, progressive disease of the lungs caused by inhaling asbestos dust or fibers).

Although he received Social Security benefits and industrial compensation, he was too handicapped to enjoy his retirement. He has sustained a total 40-pound weight loss from his youthful 165 pounds to his admission weight of 125.

Because he was coughing up blood he was admitted to the intensive care unit. The intern's history described him as an obviously chronically and seriously ill male who was extremely short of breath at rest. Laboratory tests revealed a severe anemia and serious chronic kidney disease. The chest X-ray revealed two lung tumors; in addition, there were the typical findings of emphysema and asbestosis.

A bronchoscopy revealed no tumor cells. A needle biopsy of the smaller lung tumor was performed. (The pathology report was not given to me, for part of my task was to diagnose the nature of the tumor without knowing what the pathologist diagnosed.)

Mechanical respiratory assistance was instituted for the treatment of the patient's shortness of breath. There was little improvement.

As surgical removal of the lung tumors was impossible, he was started on radiation treatments. These had to be stopped after the third treatment when the patient began to pass dark blood in his stools. This hemorrhage was treated with *8 units of red blood cells!*

Extensive X-ray examinations of the upper and lower digestive tracts failed to reveal the source of bleeding. The patient was then gastroscoped (a lighted instrument was passed down the throat into the stomach) and finally colonoscoped (a lighted instrument was passed six feet up the rectum to survey the colon). Still no source of bleeding was discovered.

On the sixteenth hospital day the patient had a convulsion which lasted for three hours and required massive doses of intravenous medication for its ultimate control. The morning following the seizures he had evidence of a stroke. A lumbar puncture was done.

He was no longer able to retain fluids, due to nausea and vomiting, so he was maintained day after day with intravenous fluids, with a careful record of his "intake and output."

As no source of the gastrointestinal bleeding had been found and as the patient was continuing to pass tarry stools (though in smaller amounts), a surgical consultation was requested. X-rays of the abdominal blood vessels were obtained by injecting dye into the abdominal aorta. This, too, failed to reveal the cause of his bleeding, which stopped spontaneously during the third week in the intensive care unit.

Finally, on the twenty-fifth hospital day, the patient was transferred to a four-bed ward and in another week to a chronic hospital for what was essentially custodial care. He remained there for eleven months, when he experienced another severe gastrointestinal hemorrhage. He was brought by ambulance to the emergency room but expired within four hours in spite of 5 units of red blood cell mass. As death occurred within less than twenty-four hours of admission, the coroner was notified and an autopsy was performed.

There were three questions with which I was to deal: What kind of lung tumors were the two that were seen by X-ray? Where and what was the source of the hemorrhage? What caused the convulsion?

My challenge as the discussant was to diagnose the type of tumor without knowing what the biopsy showed, and to tell what was the source of the hemorrhage without benefit of the autopsy report. Finally, I was expected to discuss the cause of the convulsion without knowing what the brain showed at autopsy.

The purpose of all the exhausting, painful testing as seen by the staff was to reach a diagnosis which traditionally has to precede therapeutic decisions.

One of the points I shall try to make is that circumstance can make treatment *without a full* diagnosis the method of choice in some older patients.

The auditorium where I was to discuss the CPC was full. My remarks follow essentially as I gave them.

### COMMENTS ON THE CASE

"I wish to thank you for the four days that I have spent with you in the clinics and on the wards at this renowned teaching center.

"However, at this final meeting I am going to abuse your

hospitality and 'read you a lecture' instead of discussing the patient's diagnosis, as is customary at a clinical pathological conference.

"The source of his gastrointestinal hemorrhage, the precise nature of his lung tumor, and the cause of his convulsion and subsequent weakness of left hand and forearm I will leave to the distinguished pathologists who performed the autopsy to divulge to you. To dispense with your impatience to know the final results, I will only say that the cause of the gastrointestinal hemorrhage was not discovered even at autopsy, as you know can happen, and that the convulsion and stroke were unrelated to the possible spread of lung cancer to his brain.

"Let me then, with the prerogatives accorded a guest and a person in his seventh decade, discuss with you the aspects of this case which have impressed me.

"I hope a few of my remarks to you may indeed appear in the public press. The more people outside the medical fraternity who discuss the therapeutic dilemma illustrated by this patient, the better, so far as I am concerned.

"I believe this case illustrates how, since the days of Paracelsus, William Harvey, and Ambroise Paré, we physicians, because of the impact of science and technology, have lost much of our humility and some of our humanity.

"You are taught—and I was taught—to be intolerant of any error in specific diagnosis or specific treatment while at the same time you learn to tolerate, excuse, or even overlook matters involving general judgment and general management which do not seem suitable for scientific analysis.

"I am speaking as I do because I believe this patient's experience is not rare. In fact, it is typical of what often happens in many large American teaching hospitals where the technological imperative drives medical practitioners to intervene 'because they can, not because they should.'

"The more unsophisticated the patient, the greater his risk

when the doctors in charge of his treatment, considering death an affront and a challenge, base their medical orders more on scientific facts than on value judgments and clinical impressions.

"There should be a sign on the entrance to every intensive care unit stating 'Caveat aegrotus,' which, translated, could mean 'Let the medical patient in his seventies or eighties beware!'

"I think there is general agreement that an intensive care unit is admirably suited for treating the young person suffering from a serious car or motorcycle accident. It is excellently conceived for the treatment of severe industrial and farm accidents or complicated gunshot wounds.

"It is the best place to treat the seriously and acutely ill young or middle-aged adult whose general health has always been good. It is ideal for the occasional disastrous obstetrical emergency and for the *immediate postoperative* patient of any age who has just had major surgery or a complicated or serious fracture requiring surgical intervention.

"BUT . . . in my opinion it is a very poor place for most chronically ill patients over sixty-five whose problem is medical rather than surgical!

*"I think your patient should never have been admitted to the intensive care unit.* At the very least, he should have been transferred to a two-bed room within twenty-four hours, just as soon as the multi-system chronic nature of his complicated problems became apparent.

"Let me tell you on what I base my opinion. The day after I arrived at your university I asked to see the social welfare worker's notes relevant to the patient under discussion. I wished to inform myself as completely as I could about his human situation. The following information comes from the report of your social worker who was asked to find a bed for him when he was discharged to your chronic hospital, which, in California, we call by the euphemistic phrase 'convalescent hospital.'

"Whatever the name, they are all chiefly nursing homes for incurable patients who are senile or total invalids, or both.

"I discovered that your patient was a bachelor. He had no known next of kin. He had signed the usual Conditions of Admission form, giving his written permission for 'the examinations, treatment and medications ordered by any staff physician,' *without,* I am sure, understanding the implications of this document.

"I found that prior to this patient's first visit to your outpatient clinic at age sixty-one when he developed congestive heart failure, his activities had been chiefly sitting in the lobby of the small, cheap hotel where he lived, watching television. Before he became too short of breath, he would occasionally walk to the close-by river and fish off the dock. At the time the patient was admitted to your intensive care unit, he appeared to the hotel desk clerk to be a dying man. A social worker had already been assigned to him because the hotel was unwilling to continue to rent him a room. Because the patient had visited a friend in a nursing home, he dreaded them, and had put off institutionalization from week to week.

"It seemed to me, both from the medical protocol you sent me and from the social worker's notes, that by the time this patient was admitted to your intensive care unit he was exactly what the hotel clerk thought him to be—a dying man. 'Is morbid academic curiosity a sufficiently good reason'[18] for all the tests this patient underwent after it was known that he had chronic incurable disease of the heart, of the lungs, of the kidneys?

"As I read all the diagnostic tests and therapeutic maneuvers I gasped at the wild abuse and overuse of technology in treating this patient. Although he was only sixty-three chronologically, he was obviously nearer eighty physiologically. I believe that as soon as the chest X-ray, which was available twenty-four hours after his admission, showed inoperable pulmonary carcinoma, this patient should have been transferred to a two-bed room and kept comfortable by minimal medication. By 'comfortable,' I mean both physically and emotionally, and not subjected to any of the purely academically interesting procedures which are outlined in the protocol.

"I believe—and a majority of intensive care unit nurses with whom I have spoken believe—that for the most part the intensive care unit is a poor place for the *medical* patient over sixty-five. Somehow we must learn, you and I, that even the most seriously ill medical patient does not have to be placed on an intensive care unit and be subjected to exhausting diagnostic procedures just because these units and these tests are available!

"A teaching institution such as yours has to lead the way in instructing younger doctors when NOT TO ORDER these tests and treatments. The public press must teach the public NOT TO EXPECT, NOT TO REQUIRE, NOT TO DEMAND of us, the aggressive technological approach which so often ends with only the prolongation of the functions of the patient's bodily organs and tissues, NOT HIS LIFE! I believe natural selection is often better able to decide survival than unrestrained science, particularly in the patient over sixty-five.

"Dr. Pedro A. Poma, of the Mt. Sinai Hospital Medical Center in Chicago, has emphasized that 'physicians are limited in their abilities to improve people's health'; that people have an 'overly optimistic view of the potential of medical science.'[19] I agree with Dr. Poma's conclusion that you and I must emphasize to our patients the limitations of medicine."

# Chapter 9

## A Call for Consultation

It seems to me that medicine should consider the possibility of contributing more by doing less.

Victor Fuchs, Ph.D., in *The Western Journal of Medicine,* July 1976

### A SUDDEN CRISIS

My secretary, who is an R.N., has held down the front desk for fifteen years. She never disturbs me when I am talking to a patient unless the matter is urgent.

"Helen is calling from the Los Angeles airport. She seems upset and wants to see you this afternoon to talk about her mother. Your appointment book is full, Dr. Baer."

Helen is the person you met in Chapter 1.

"Tell her to catch the next plane to San Francisco and come directly to the office. Have sandwiches sent in. She and I can have our lunch here and talk."

Helen waited for me to finish my sandwich and then started talking.

"It's Mother again. She's developed what her doctor calls a small pregangrenous ulcer on her right great toe. For years she wore her shoes too small and the second toe encroaches on the great toe. The nurses have tried to keep lamb's wool between the toes to relieve the pressure, but the ulcer is slowly growing in diameter and depth and has become painful. The problem is made worse, her doctor says, by her poor circulation. For several years he has not been able to feel a pulse in either foot.

"In addition, Mother has been in and out of congestive heart failure the past two years in spite of maximum doses of digitalis and diuretics. So, there is no chance her foot will heal unless further steps are taken; in fact, the doctor says the ulcer will soon expose the underlying tendon and bone.

"A vascular surgeon saw Mother in consultation and recommends she be transferred back to the hospital for a lumbar sympathectomy [cutting the nerves in the interior of the low abdomen in the hope of increasing the circulation in the leg]. He thinks this may improve the blood flow to the lower leg and permit the ulcer to heal.

"If it does not, he recommends amputation, either of the toe or the foot. Otherwise, he says the pain will increase as the ulcer enlarges.

"My sister and I want you to fly to Los Angeles to see Mother in consultation. Both doctors agree. Mother of course does not understand anything at all. She just complains of pain and asks when she can go home.

"Will you see her?"

I answered that I would fly down on Sunday. "If one or both of the other doctors could meet me after I have examined your mother, we could hold a consultation and advise you and your sister of our recommendations."

Helen made the arrangements. She and Dan and I took the 9:30 A.M. plane to Los Angeles. Her sister met us at the airport and drove us to the convalescent hospital. We arrived just after 11 o'clock. The other two doctors said they would try to be there close to noon.

The substance of the patient's medical history and the consultation follows.

## CONSULTATION NOTES

### MEDICAL CONSULTATION
### ON MRS. JOYCE DOUGLAS, AGE EIGHTY-SEVEN

Date _____

This patient is seen in consultation at the request of her two daughters and with the approval of her attending physician, J. W. Ray, M.D.

The patient is a frail, 87-year-old woman appearing chronically ill and slightly short of breath at rest.

*Chief Complaints*—(1) "My foot hurts"; (2) "I want to go home."

*Present Illness*—She believes her foot has hurt a "long time" but cannot say how long or how it began. Yes, it does interfere with sleep. There is relief from the shots the nurse gives her; she cannot estimate the duration of the relief.

When asked where her home is, she says "Kansas."

When asked who would care for her at home, she says "my daughter."

*Limited Physical Examination*
Pulse 92; Resp. 18; Blood Pressure 180/70
The positive findings are:
*Neurologic*—She was tested twice by means of the Cognitive Capacity Test[20] [an intelligence test for patients with severe brain damage], and scored zero out of 30. She did not know the day of the week, the month, or the year. She could not give the opposite of "up" or "large" or "hard." She could not complete

the sentence, "Red and blue are both _____," or "A penny and a dime are both _____."

She gave her name, but as to her age or date of birth, said, "I do not know." She could not give Helen's married name, nor her son-in-law's first name.

When asked if there was anything a doctor could do for her, she answered, "Yes, get me out of here!"

*Cardiovascular*—The heart is fibrillating and enlarged; the murmurs of mitral stenosis and insufficiency are easily heard; pulses are absent in both feet and the legs blanched with elevation.

*Ulcer*—There is a superficial, chronic-appearing ulcer on the medial lateral surface of the right great toe. It measures ½ cm. in diameter and 1 mm. in depth. There is no evidence of healing.

*Conclusion*—This patient is suffering from chronic, incurable progressive, far-advanced disease of her brain, heart, and peripheral blood vessels. She has a small, nonhealing pre-gangrenous ulcer of the right great toe.

### Discussion

While a successful sympathectomy might promote the healing of her ulcer, it would subject her to the additional physical and emotional distress of being transferred to the hospital, being prepared for major surgery, undergoing general anesthesia, etc. Even if this ulcer healed, her fundamental incapacitating brain and heart disease would be unaltered.

Subjecting her to possible amputation is even less desirable, in my opinion, from the patient's point of view.

I therefore cannot agree with Dr. Lyon's recommendation of sympathectomy and possible amputation.

Rather, I am in favor of:

(1) Transferring her home (as she ardently wishes). An electrical hospital bed can be rented and placed in her daughter's living room;

(2) Providing round-the-clock nursing—her two daughters plus a licensed vocational nurse for night duty;

(3) Increasing the dose of Demerol so that she obtains at least

6 hours' relief of pain, anxiety, and shortness of breath, and in
addition

(4) Using Demerol liberally for sleep and its euphorogenic quali-
ties;

(5) Discontinuing the chemical prolongation of the action of
her dying heart by stopping her digitalis and Dyazide, without which I would anticipate natural death from heart failure
in two weeks.

It is quite apparent to me that without these two drugs this
totally senile patient would have died nearly two and a half years
ago and been spared the nursing home incarceration and the
ulcer which has come to plague her. I think further scientific
chemical prolongation of her biologic existence even by these
standard drugs is no longer justifiable.

I will discuss these opinions and my advice with her family
and attending physician.

[Signed] L.S.B.


When I had finished examining Mrs. Douglas and writing my
consultation notes in her chart I joined Helen, her sister, and
Dan in the small nursing home reception room.

"It is customary for a consultant not to discuss his findings
or opinion with members of the family until after he has talked
privately with the attending physician. I'll wait here for the
other doctors while you go out for a quick lunch. You may join
us as soon as we have had a chance to reach an agreement on
the advice we will offer you."


## THE DOCTORS' CONSULTATION

Shortly thereafter, Dr. Ray, the attending physician (a man
in his mid-fifties), arrived with Dr. Lyon (the vascular surgeon,
who appeared to be in his late thirties).

I introduced myself and asked them to be kind enough to read my consultation notes.

Dr. Lyon was the first to speak. "With all respect to you, Dr. Baer, and your forty years of practice and your academic rank, I disagree. If your plan is followed, I will have to dissociate myself from any responsibility for the patient and I will feel compelled so to state my feelings in her chart.

"In all my years of practice I never heard of such a recommendation being made, let alone followed. What it amounts to is giving up all efforts to help the patient or improve her condition and just letting her die."

I listened while Dr. Ray spoke up. "I have cared for Mrs. Douglas for ten years, Dr. Baer, and watched her slowly and inexorably go downhill. She can't go down much farther and she can't go on much longer. I would appreciate your thoughts on the medical ethics of the course you recommend. I think the purely scientific and pathologic facts are clear to each of us."

"I am sure, gentlemen, what each of us wants is to be of help to this patient. It is understandable that we should differ as to how to do that. For my part, Dr. Lyon, I have the highest regard for your skill and surgical judgment. Let me, if I can, take you step by step along the path of thinking that led to my recommendations.

"The patient is an old lady who has already survived, according to the history in her chart, open-heart surgery, at age fifty-two. This saved her life and gave her thirty-five extra years of good living. Three times since age eighty-one, she has been in acute congestive heart failure and by prompt medical treatment improved. The first two times she was able to go back to the apartment where she lived happily with her daughter. The last time when she had the nearly fatal stroke, her life was saved, but she had to come here where she has been for two and a half years. She was just too much of a nursing problem for her daughter, who worked a full forty-hour week.

"So, four times medicine and surgery have extended her life; the quality of that life was good until the last episode.

"Now her brain is so damaged she can't tell you much, but what she does say is clear enough: (1) the 'toe hurts'; (2) she wants 'to go home,' i.e., she does not want to stay where she is.

"Further, though she cannot say so, I am sure she is like each of us. When our time comes to die, if it's to be from a chronic illness, we all would prefer to be in our bed at home, attended only by those we have loved and recognized and to have someone at hand during our actual dying moments.

"None of this is possible for her in the nursing home.

"Nor, because of the full-time nursing needs, is this possible for a long time at her old apartment. But for a short time it is quite possible. If she could speak, I believe this lady would say that she does not want, above all, to have her act of dying chemically and scientifically prolonged—which is precisely what the 'routine' daily doses of digitalis and diuretics are doing.

"What do I mean by a 'short time'? I mean precisely the length of time it would take her to die a natural death from natural causes, eased of anxiety and physical distress by Demerol, but not prolonged one more day by the powerful diuretics that modern chemistry has made available.

"I feel profoundly that science has done as much as it can for this patient. I believe now it is the time for humanity to speak forcefully and let her die in peace, quickly and naturally, and in her own bed.

"I rather suspect that the joy of arriving back home will be the greatest felicity she has known in the past two and a half years.

"Medically, it is clear that though the ulcer might slowly heal following a successful sympathectomy, that outcome is not at all certain; and then she is faced with amputation of the toe or the foot. Even if it did heal, her brain and heart would continue to get worse."

Dr. Ray spoke up. "As the attending physician, I would like to make a few observations before we meet with Mrs. Douglas' daughters.

"Because of her senility she really has no way of making her own choice as to whether or not she wants to prolong her existence by continuing her digitalis and powerful diuretics. She only takes the medicine now because the nurses stand by her bedside, put them in her mouth, and watch her swallow them. . . .

"I agree medically with Dr. Baer that because of the extraordinary effectiveness of our modern diuretics she may go on as she is for six months or a year or more. I am therefore willing to concur in your judgment."

"If you will permit me one final word," I interrupted, "I believe some of the difference in approach to this patient's management between Dr. Lyon and myself is that during his surgical training he followed his patients through their postoperative recovery, but he has not had the learning opportunity afforded a family doctor of following that same patient for several years. The immediate postoperative results of surgery on the elderly are often different from the long-term results in quality of their life."

I went outside, found Helen, her sister, and Dan waiting, and asked them to join us.

Dr. Ray acted as our spokesman.

"We have discussed Dr. Baer's recommendation for Mrs. Douglas. From the surgical point of view, Dr. Lyon disagrees with our conclusions and asks not to be included in the plan that Dr. Baer and I favor. You two sisters will have to be the ones to decide.

"To be brief, Dr. Lyon recommends your mother be readmitted to the hospital for a sympathectomy in the hope that this will improve the circulation to her foot and permit the ulcer to heal.

"If this fails, he then recommends amputation of the toe or the foot sufficiently high to encounter healthy tissue.

"Dr. Baer and I think that your mother has over a lifetime derived much benefit from medical and surgical science. But now we perceive that any further continuation of scientific medicine will only prolong her physical and mental suffering, not relieve it.

"We are making a *distinctly unusual*—but we feel quite ethical and moral—recommendation. We believe that the most loving and reasonable step is to STOP all 'existence-prolonging' measures, namely, her digitalis and her powerful diuretics; obtain a hospital bed and engage an L.V.N., and send your mother home! We think Mrs. Weinstein, who I understand is a retired R.N., can take a daytime shift and a competent L.V.N. can take the evening shift. If you, Miss Douglas, obtain leave of absence from your job, then your mother will receive personal care not obtainable anywhere else. Demerol will be prescribed both by mouth and by hypodermic to relieve any pain, shortness of breath, sleeplessness, or anxiety.

"We fully anticipate that Mrs. Douglas will die a natural death from heart failure within ten days or two weeks after returning home. Dr. Baer, do you have anything to add to what I have said?"

"No, Dr. Ray, I think the family should discuss our recommendations privately. If they want further consultation, I am sure we three would welcome it."

Three days later Helen called me from Los Angeles to say that she, Dan, and her sister had gone to the hospital where her mother had been a patient on the two last occasions her heart had failed. They spoke to the hospital chaplain who had visited her.

He felt the advice they had received was compassionate and correct from the point of view of a woman who no longer could be said to be "holding on to life," if by life was meant the total human being—body, mind, and spirit. Rather, he felt that total life had already been extinguished and that what remained was an artificially supported existence of the body.

Her mother had been brought home today and was resting quietly. Dr. Ray had ordered an ample supply of Demerol and told them to use it liberally as needed.

Mrs. Douglas did indeed die quietly during the afternoon ten days later with both her daughters in attendance.

## POSTSCRIPT

The final event was a letter to me from Dr. Ray in mid-June saying he had been asked to appear before his county medical society's ethics committee to discuss the case—would I come down that day and appear with him?

I would and I did!

The committee, composed of fourteen of our peers, voted to approve of our management of this difficult moral problem.

The vote was 8 in favor of our action, 4 opposed, and 2 abstaining.

# Part Two
# Toward
# a Solution

(Ways to Avoid Dying in a Nursing Home)

Worn-out garments are shed
by the body. Worn-out bodies
are shed by the dweller
within the body.

**Bhagavad-Gita**

# Chapter 10

## Your Most
## Important Decision

> We have perverted the Judeo-Christian tradition into a belief that biological existence *per se* is of supreme value, and on the basis of that interpretation have been sidetracked into an ethical dilemma of ghastly proportions.
>
> Rev. Robert B. Reeves, Jr., First
> Euthanasia Conference, Nov. 23, 1968

Practically everyone, if given the choice, would avoid years of senility and invalidism in a long-term-care institution. This is true even of persons who have never visited a convalescent hospital or nursing home. Such institutions, however, are an expanding enterprise on the American scene. Each year more and more of them are appearing. New facilities are increasingly larger, better equipped, and more expensive. The number of their occupants is increasing as well as the total number of months or years each patient stays. That's why nursing homes are considered a good investment!

Statistics can be cited to show the success of modern medicine and surgery in shortening the usual hospital stay by several days. What is not explained is that they have increased the number of older persons needing nursing home care and have prolonged the average stay in nursing homes by many months or years.

## LIFE IN A NURSING HOME

Many long-term-care institutions publish attractive brochures describing their adult education classes, live musical entertainment, field trips, parties, games, and companionship. But the percentage of residents who could possibly participate in such programs is only a small minority, perhaps 15 percent of the total number.

Over my lifetime of practice in one community I have visited almost all the long-term-care institutions in the area. What I have observed in these institutions would, I believe, hold true for similar institutions in other parts of the country. Many of the better nursing homes are well equipped, and have attractive, well-maintained buildings. They are staffed by competent, hardworking, *underpaid,* and compassionate personnel. They are doing as well as anyone could expect with a virtually impossible task.

Most of the patients in such a facility are almost totally incapable of caring for themselves. They need to be taken from place to place; they need to be dressed, bathed, taken to the toilet, and fed by others. Their medicines must be administered on schedule, with the nurse responsible that the pills are actually swallowed. When all these attentions have been properly charted in each patient's record, it is time to rebathe the incontinent, change the beds, reapply the posey belts to restrain those who would fall or wander away if left entirely on their own.

In addition to the care of patients, nursing home personnel are required by law to complete a mountain of triplicate forms for every patient; and the next mail brings more forms, always with an imminent deadline requiring signatures from doctors, family, suppliers, and government officials. These are some of the reasons I feel nursing home personnel are among the hardest-working and most underpaid personnel in the whole medical profession.

It is the patients who most depress any visitor to a nursing home. To see them slumped in the corridors or in the TV room —one hundred or two hundred per institution, many of them unable to respond to the simplest question, much less go on a field trip or play games—is to behold the agony of dying indefinitely prolonged. One immediately concurs with Mrs. Lillian Carter, who says, "I'm glad I worked at the Nursing Home, but God forbid that I ever have to live in one!"[21]

In the poorer nursing homes the situation is predictably worse. The ratio of patients to staff is higher; therefore the overload is greater. Even the most compassionate nurses and nurses aides will find their patience and benevolence worn thin after a time, despite their best intentions. I believe the custom that primitive nomadic tribes had of leaving the elderly disabled behind was more humane by far than our scientifically oriented institutional methods of dealing with them.

It is not surprising, therefore, that *all* my older patients are agreed about what they most dread. It is not the fear of death, but the dread of becoming demented, or totally dependent, and then being confined in an extended care facility. And I strongly suspect that my patients are no different in this regard from older people generally. No one wants to be a non-person, a burden and a care in old age. But how can it reasonably be avoided?

## SOME PEOPLE LIVE LONG, HEALTHY LIVES

If you wish to die young as old as possible, it is more important to have good genes than a good doctor. I am sure that we doctors, with only seventy-five years of experience in scientific medicine to guide us, often are not as capable of deciding how long a patient should live as nature is.

The DNA double helix which makes each of us what we are took millions of years to develop. The forty-six chromosomes and the millions of genes which have been shaped by our fore-bears are a powerful determinant of how long one is likely to live in vigorous good health. Thus, in simple terms, if your ancestors were inclined to longevity and good health, your chances of sharing the same are greatly enchanced. But since we had noth-ing to do with choosing our ancestors, this means of avoiding spending our last years in a nursing home lies beyond our con-trol.

Some of the things, however, that contribute to good health and longevity are within our control. Proper eating and exercise and faithful disciplines of hygiene are important throughout life. Preventive medicine through regular visits to doctor and dentist may allow early diagnosis of remedial health problems. Such practices should probably not be neglected as one advances in age.

Smoking is also something that we can control if that hap-pens to be a habit. I am not referring just now to the relationship of smoking to cancer. A friend of mine who is an emergency room doctor says that most of the patients he sees under age sixty-five who have had a heart attack, or those under age seventy who have had a stroke, are heavy smokers. Beyond age sixty-five, a male who smokes heavily ages ten years faster than a non-smoking female. Admittedly, a lifelong habit is difficult to break. It can be done, but wishing won't make it so. A firm commitment of will to stop smoking could add healthy years to the life of a heavy smoker.

## AGING IS INEVITABLE

We begin growing older from the moment of birth. Certainly the first years of life have a maturing dimension. We reach our physical peak normally in our early twenties, and most people remain healthy and vigorous for the next thirty or forty years. But aging is inevitably taking place. It is of no use to pretend at the age of sixty-five that we are still thirty or forty. Cardiovascular ailments occur far more frequently in persons in their sixties and seventies than when they are one or two decades younger.

A friend who is a cardiologist made the sensible observation that if a person's coronary arteries are diseased at age sixty-five, so too in varying degrees are his arteries to the brain and probably to the legs and kidneys as well.

The older one's body becomes, the less resilient it is to injury and disease. Since modern methods of treating serious ailments place severe stress upon the whole system, the result for older patients can be miraculous or incapacitating. Biological life may be preserved, but multiple debilitating side effects of the illness or the treatment continue indefinitely.

Coronary bypass surgery certainly can improve the quality, if not the length, of life for a man of forty-five or fifty-five who has increasingly severe and incapacitating attacks of angina pectoris (chest pain due to decreased blood supply to the heart muscle). But for the man of sixty-five or seventy-five, the desirability of this popular operation (whose proper place will take more time to evaluate) is more difficult to assess.

Many a thoughtful patient in his eighth decade of life may decide for himself that the threat of a sudden death from a heart attack (implicit where there is exceedingly severe angina) might be far preferable to the morbidity that can result from X-raying the heart's blood vessels and undergoing bypass heart surgery.

He might well conclude that for him after a full life, death from a massive heart attack (which is one of the best ways I know to die) is preferable by far to slow disintegration. I believe it is far better for the heart to go before the brain!

A man or woman of seventy or more should have to die but once. *If you "will it so,"* and are ready to forgo the possibility of a medical miracle, that once can be quick or relatively brief.

This may well be the most important decision of your later years. See what your doctor thinks about this.

## SENILITY—THE INCURABLE
## SCOURGE OF THE OLD

The medical terms describing senility include: incapacitating senility, senile dementia, severe organic brain disease, advanced cerebral atrophy, serious arteriosclerotic brain disease, hardening of the arteries to the brain, or simply senility. They all mean the same—severe impairment of the blood supply to the brain due to hardening of the arteries that nourish it. Brain cells then die and, rapidly or slowly at age fifty, sixty, seventy, eighty, or ninety, the patient progressively loses his memory, ability to read, write, calculate, and care for himself.

We do not know why some people are afflicted early in life and some never, or not until their mid-nineties.

The cause of hardening of the arteries to the brain is still a mystery, although there are more than one hundred theories. The cure is still unknown, although a thousand treatments have been tried. We know many factors that play a role in senility, but the fundamental cause eludes us. Certainly smoking in excess, a diet high in saturated fats, and high blood pressure statistically predispose to cerebral arteriosclerosis.

In many cases senility is far more progressive, relentless, incurable, and incapacitating than cancer. It is indeed an untreatable and progressive disease.

It could afflict me, my wife, or *you* at any time!

The advanced senile patient is more of a nursing problem than ninety-nine out of one hundred private homes can manage. They are demented and wander unless restrained; they wet themselves, soil themselves, constantly fall, babble, and are totally dependent on others for bathing, dressing, feeding, toilet needs, and sometimes walking or even sitting up!

An important fact to remember is that tens of thousands of senile patients in nursing homes are there because, prior death from natural causes (in an older patient already infirm) was prevented by aggressive medicine or surgery, or simply because *ordinary, everyday* modern drugs are so very powerful.

When I was in medical school, if a senile patient needed a catheter to keep him from being wet with urine all day and night, the catheter would inevitably cause a severe urinary tract infection. Then in a few weeks at the most, this would lead to kidney infection, to kidney failure and a quiet death in a few months.

Today, you *cannot* die of a urinary tract infection. Two or three sulfa tablets a day is all it takes to prevent natural death for years. And if sulfa does not work, we have half a dozen more powerful urinary antiseptics.

The same is true of pneumonia. Senile patients in nursing homes frequently died quickly of pneumonia in the 1930's. Not today! It would be malpractice!

Antibiotics are not heroic or extraordinary treatments. *But they are very powerful and effective in killing bacteria.* Tens of thousands of grossly senile patients are prevented from dying a natural death by daily routine prophylactic urinary antibiotics, administered in the name of "good medical practice."

Forty years ago, nursing home patients frequently died of heart failure—not today! Ordinary modern diuretics (drugs that cause the body to excrete in the urine any excess fluid that has accumulated because of heart failure) are very powerful. Given in pill form once or twice a day, in conjunction with a digitalis, they can and regularly do prevent death from congestive heart failure for *years!*

Aging for all is an inevitable fact of life, and senility in varying degrees an affliction of many in their later years. Why try to pretend such things do not happen, or will never happen to you? Far better it is to face reality while you can. There are specific things you can and should do.

## WHY NOT FACE IT NOW?

To borrow a technique from Gautama Buddha, who was certainly one of the most successful teachers of all the ages, here is the sixfold path leading away from a nursing home:

*Inform yourself* of the avoidable human causes that can lead to a nursing home existence for yourself.

*Question yourself* as to what you want from modern medicine and what you don't want.

*Ask your doctor* for his advice.

*Discuss the matter* with your family or closest friend.

*Decide what you are willing* to forgo medically in order to avoid scientific prolongation of your existence.

*Act* on the choice you make.

Assuming that the first five seem reasonable enough, what is involved in step six?

Let me tell you what I have done for myself and what I recommend to all my patients who are over sixty-five and who are determined *not* to end their life in an extended care facility.

### THE MEDIC-ALERT TAG

A medical or surgical disaster could easily strike you far from home. If the illness or injury was so severe as to prevent communication of thoughts and ability to speak for yourself, you would be rushed to the nearest emergency room and the medical system would go to work.

There would be no way that the doctors and the nurses could know your wishes, and heroic efforts of every type would be made, *and maintained,* to continue the function of your vital organs no matter how old you are or how serious the injury or illness. You might attach a negative value to such efforts, but who would know?

To make my own wishes known in such an eventuality I always wear a Medic-Alert bracelet[22] (my wife wears a tag on a pendant around her neck).

My wife's and mine say:


Line 1 <u>POSITIVELY NO</u>

Line 2 <u>RESUSCITATION.</u>

Line 3 <u>NO I.V.   NO INJ.</u>

Line 4 <u>NO INTUBATION.</u>


The bracelet speaks for you if your brain is so damaged or diseased that you cannot speak for yourself. If you do not like the phraseology, devise your own with the aid of your doctor.

Naturally, if you are alert at the time of a serious accident or illness, you can always discuss your treatment with your doctor. But if you are so seriously ill or injured that you cannot communicate your thoughts, then your Medic-Alert tag does it for you, 24 hours a day, 365 days a year!

Translated, the bracelet says that if you suffer a catastrophic illness or injury which so severely damages your brain's capacity to function that you cannot communicate your thoughts, then, in case of cardiopulmonary arrest, lines 1 and 2 say *you positively forbid* ANY attempts at resuscitation which might well start your heart beating and restart your breathing but leave you with your brain permanently incapacitated. Doctors classify patients with brain damage as having a severe, moderate, or what is euphemistically called *"only* a mild organic brain syndrome" where just one or two, instead of all or many, of the brain functions are damaged.

Well I, for one, do not choose to be resuscitated and have "only" mild brain damage. I am appalled at such a thought! I plan to avoid it AT ALL COSTS for myself if that is within my power. The older a patient is, the more quickly the brain cells die from lack of oxygen! The brain is at its peak of physiologic perfection at age twenty-four.

Line 3 of the bracelet *forbids* intravenous fluids or medicine (I.V.) in an attempt to revive you or to keep you alive; and line 3 further *forbids* any and all injections (INJ.) to try to do the same.

I am adamant about this because, having seen much organic brain disease in adults due to trauma, surgery, and disease, I have a horror of it which I do not have for a sudden or quick death.

The last line (line 4) *prohibits* tubes (INTUBATION) of any type being inserted into the trachea so that the respiratory assistance apparatus can be hooked up! It can be started by any authorized person, but no one dares to turn it off!

These rules permit a rapid, natural death. They preclude my being kept alive to die more slowly, lingering for years in an institution because of enthusiastic, aggressive, scientific, and technical treatments. It leaves the outcome up to nature, which is where I want it!

We are members of the species *Homo sapiens.* When we are no longer sapient, no matter what the cause, we should be permitted to die a natural death with only good nursing care, pain relief and sedation, and no scientific medicine.

Naturally, the wording on my Medic-Alert tag, which is precisely what I wish, may not be what you would wish and might not be what your doctor would recommend. You can use any phraseology on your Medic-Alert tag that you wish to inform medical personnel everywhere at all times what are your specific desires.

There is room for fourteen letters on each of the four lines. You might prefer a less positive statement than I chose. For example:

Line 1 <u>POSITIVELY NO</u>

Line 2 <u>RESUSCITATION</u>

Line 3 <u>LONGER THAN</u>

Line 4 <u>TWO MINUTES.</u>*

*or FIVE MINUTES, if your doctor concurs.

Even a Medic-Alert bracelet can be overlooked or even ignored!

I showed mine to one of our keen young cardiologists who has seen several of my patients in consultation and has always been helpful to them and to me. I asked him if I were brought into the emergency room in cardiopulmonary arrest and he was on duty and he saw my bracelet, what would he do?

He answered: "I would probably attempt to resuscitate you anyway. You might have been depressed the day you put the bracelet on"!

As you can see from this personal anecdote, both doctors and patients have much to learn about:

the formation,
the transmittal,
and *the following out* of a competent patient's "orders."

I do not advocate that a patient tell the doctor how to treat an ailment. Rather, I am trying to suggest practical means whereby the cognizant patient can *order* that certain modalities of therapy are *not to be used* under specific circumstances.

Most doctors could welcome such help from their patients, for today scientific medical decisions are hard enough without we physicians having also to bear moral and ethical decisions which are not our prerogative and duty to make.

I am sure a *modus vivendi* can be worked out to permit hospitalized patients to play an increasingly knowledgeable and responsible role in making these awesome decisions about their only life and their only death.

I decided to outline my personal approach to this problem, because it seems to me that at present the "scientific imperative" frequently takes precedence over the patient's all too often unexpressed wishes.

To do the best for our patients, we doctors truly need formal patient's orders.

# Chapter 11

## Confronting Major Afflictions

The proper function of man is to live, not to exist.

Jack London, from I. Shepard (ed.),
*Jack London's Tales of Adventure*

As one advances in years the incidence of major ailments increases. We have already noted that some people live long and remarkably healthy lives. When this is the case, hereditary factors appear to be the major reason that it is so. There is surely some correlation between proper diet, exercise, and personal hygiene and the general state of one's health and well-being. Still, major afflictions of one type or another are likely to confront most of us in our lifetime, and they do come more frequently as we grow older.

To be able to face the future realistically, it is necessary to understand as much as we can about the ailments that are likely to beset us in our later years. Therefore, in this chapter I wish to describe the afflictions that older persons do confront, and to assess in realistic terms the problems and limitations that they impose. What real threat do they hold for ending one's days in an extended care facility, and under what circumstances can that eventuality be avoided?

## WHAT ABOUT A HEART ATTACK?

The medical problem that a person age sixty-five is most likely to face in the next five years is a "sudden heart attack" or "coronary." The medical term is myocardial infarction (MI). This common affliction is caused by a blood clot in one of the coronary arteries (the blood vessels that supply the heart muscle itself). The blood clot prevents blood from reaching that part of the heart which it supplies and therefore this heart muscle dies.

A large majority of patients over sixty-five make a good recovery from their first myocardial infarction, no matter where or how they are treated. Actually the man who has his first "coronary" at sixty-five has a better chance of making a good recovery than the man who has his first attack at age thirty-five. That's because by the seventh decade of life you have developed many small collateral blood vessels and the heart muscle can be partially nourished by these if there is an obstruction to one of its larger arteries. This situation is analogous to the many branches of an older tree.

It is also true that your prognosis, in the case of a heart attack, is better if you do not smoke, are easygoing, have normal blood pressure, exercise regularly, and do not have diabetes or high blood pressure, or a very markedly elevated blood cholesterol or triglyceride level.

In Chapter 6, I discussed the general arrangement and operation of a modern coronary care unit. Its chief purpose is to attempt instantaneous correction of potentially fatal abnormal heart rate or rhythm, which frequently complicates a myocardial infarction. There is no question of the potential benefit of this to a patient of sixty-five.

The other chief purpose of the coronary care unit is to attempt immediate resuscitation in the case of cardiac and respiratory arrest. It is this feature of the coronary care unit which, I believe, requires careful consideration by the potential coronary patient over sixty-five.

It is obvious that any decision you may make regarding treatment of a coronary occlusion that may occur to you must *precede* the attack, for at the time the pain actually comes a lot of pressure builds up instantly. It is akin to the awful moment you are first awakened from sleep by the rumble and movement by a 6.0 Richter scale earthquake. A true coronary occlusion is an awesome event.

We need not consider here the instantaneously fatal coronary occlusion which occurs either during your sleep or at some time when you are by yourself and beyond assistance.

What we need to consider is the average coronary occlusion occurring in a person over sixty-five who has time to call for assistance. Just by surviving long enough to call for help, your statistical chances of recovering are about 80 percent if this is your first attack and you are in good general health. The best equipped and staffed coronary care units may give you another 5 percent additional chance of ultimate survival.

Statistics vary depending upon which hospital group they come from, which group of patients are being reported, and which doctor or group of doctors is making the report.

Last year a report from England concerning patients over sixty-five affirmed that the patients treated at home had a better chance of survival than the ones treated in the coronary care unit.[23] My cardiology colleagues naturally do not concur with these findings. The point I am trying to emphasize is that your survival from a coronary occlusion is in large measure determined by chance. How large a blood vessel is plugged with the clot, which blood vessel it is, what was the state of your heart and general health before the occlusion, how much collateral circulation you already have, and other factors. The ultimate outcome *is not totally* related to whether or not you are admitted to a modern coronary care unit for treatment.

In general, I feel that the healthy patient between sixty-five and seventy derives some benefit from the preventive medicine features of the CCU. If a potentially fatal heart rhythm can be prevented by the proper administration of drugs or instantly treated should it develop, this I account good medicine.

But what each patient over sixty-five must consider with his doctor and then with himself and his family, is the built-in heroic resuscitation efforts that are mandatory on all coronary care units.

I recently had a chance to discuss this matter with one of the most distinguished internists on the West Coast. I have known him well for thirty years. He has an international reputation in the field of abnormal heart rate and rhythm. He is a physician's physician, the man whom doctors consult for their own family's serious medical problems. He is called when doctors disagree among themselves as to the proper diagnosis or treatment of a complicated case. In brief, a man universally respected by his colleagues and peers. He is sixty-seven years old and active in practice, teaching, and research.

I asked him this question: "What if you were a patient on a coronary care unit and you suffered a cardiorespiratory arrest two days after a moderately severe coronary occlusion? How long would you want efforts made to resuscitate you?" He answered without the slightest hesitation: "Two minutes and no more!" I agree!

A substantial majority of internists between sixty-five and seventy years of age would limit cardiopulmonary resuscitation on themselves to 2–5 minutes, not the usual 20–30 minute attempt.

The decision is yours. It involves opinion and value judgment as well as facts.

As for myself, my doctor and my family know that I forbid anything whatsoever beyond two minutes. If in that length of time I do not have a viable heart rhythm and spontaneous respiration, I forbid any further measures. If I am resuscitated in two minutes, I believe the chances of brain damage to be insignificant.

Each person must decide this difficult question for himself. Every five years beyond sixty-five makes brain damage due to a brief cardiac arrest more likely. Other illnesses complicating the myocardial infarction make good recovery less likely. A previous serious myocardial infarction makes resuscitation from a second infarction much more hazardous both from the standpoint of brain damage and heart muscle damage.

To choose what treatment you desire, you must know the facts. You must also understand the way your doctor feels about you. And most clearly, you must understand how you feel about your own act of dying. Certainly, there is a point in everyone's life at which time one would gladly accept sudden death rather than hazard uncertain resuscitation with a damaged brain.

I cannot decide this for anyone but myself. All I can do is stimulate you to think about it and make your own decision and make this decision known where it will count. For if you don't, and if you are admitted to a coronary care unit without previously discussing both the Yin as well as the Yang with your doctor, the system will take over. You will be assured of heroic, all-out efforts to maintain the beating of your heart to the very end and beyond! If that's what you want, fine. It will be delivered expertly. If that's not what you want, say it while you can, before the crisis.

Your doctor has complete authority, both ethically and legally, to limit a resuscitation attempt to any time that you and he agree is suitable to your case. But he won't be able to discuss it with you when you are sick. And you won't be able to understand him or help him reach a decision. You must think about it while you are well and discuss it with him while you have the time. There does not even have to be an attempt to resuscitate you if this is what you desire, and this is what he agrees to. I am certain there are many patients in their eighties, or whose lives have been complicated by other illnesses, who would prefer no resuscitation. This is no problem so long as you tell your doctor, for he will write it on your Physician's Orders form, the order sheet concerning your care in the hospital. But he cannot write such an order unless you request and authorize him to do so. Nor will he ask you what are your wishes. He will assume that unless you bring the matter up, you wish full resuscitation attempts, no matter what.

Remember, it must be on your order sheet if that is what you want, for at the time of a cardiac arrest it is unlikely that your own doctor will be there and the nurses in charge and the doctors who happen to be in the hospital will be the ones to take action. The only thing that will prevent them from performing a full half-hour resuscitation attempt is written orders to the contrary, and those orders can come only from you to your doctor.

What are the general chances of a patient over sixty-five who undergoes resuscitation efforts on a coronary care unit? I believe that 80 percent of the attempts are total failures. The patient dies. The catastrophically damaged heart cannot be made to function. Somewhere between 5 percent and 10 percent of the attempts are variably successful. These patients make fair, good, or excellent recoveries following what would have been certain death. On the other hand, 5 percent to 10 percent of the efforts only prolong the act of dying for minutes, hours, days, weeks, or months. The decision is yours to make—the dilemma facing all of us is difficult. It has no solution—it has only an approach.

## WHAT ABOUT A STROKE?

The chance of a stroke increases each year after age sixty. So does the fear of it.

I believe that in the majority of cases of stroke, "nature heals while the physician collects the fees." Occasionally, reducing a very high blood pressure may help, but *good nursing care* is chiefly what is needed. Vascular surgery, tried frequently ten years ago, is used much less today. Too often the cerebrovascular X-rays and the surgical intervention made the patient worse. It is still used occasionally. New techniques, which are yet untested, are always being developed, but I doubt that I would ever permit a surgical approach to a stroke for myself. In the recovery phases, of course, the services of a good physiotherapist are imperative.

As for a mild stroke, you need have little concern for yourself over the outcome. The vast majority of patients of this type spontaneously make good recoveries, partial or total.

Even from a moderately severe stroke, which does not involve the language center, you can expect sufficient recovery after two or three weeks of conservative management in the hospital, and with two to three months of good nursing care at home, plus some outpatient physical therapy to avoid the necessity of a nursing home.

Naturally, you should be in an acute hospital for the first week or two after a moderate stroke to have the proper care of your toilet and bathing needs, and to start daily physical therapy.

At the other extreme of the stroke spectrum, the sudden massive catastrophic stroke, such as Franklin D. Roosevelt suffered, is of no concern as far as a nursing home is involved. This type is mercifully fatal in a few minutes, before modern medical science can intervene to prolong the person's existence.

But the stroke that so often leads directly to months or years in a convalescent hospital is the very severe but not immediately fatal one. This is the type we all fear and with good reason. Its hallmark is extensive paralysis and loss of consciousness.

However, instead of dying in a few minutes or in an hour or two, the heart continues to beat and the person continues to breathe. That is because the "vital centers" in the brain are usually the last to die—days, weeks, months, or years after the more vulnerable sentient parts. What makes this type of stroke so frightful, in my opinion, is the nearly automatic and routine ordering of intravenous fluids for the patient.

I have told my doctor that if I have a stroke and am stuporous, comatose, or have such severe aphasia (inability to speak or to understand either the spoken or the written word)—in other words, if I am not able to communicate clearly my thoughts to my doctor—I positively forbid him to keep me alive with intravenous fluids even for six hours, let alone six days.

Intravenous glucose is *standard* treatment and not considered aggressive or heroic by any means. It is routine to start an intravenous on any patient who has had a stroke and cannot swallow liquids. Because it is standard practice is the precise reason I have forbidden my doctor to start the intravenous on me if I have such a stroke. The worst final results of stroke that I have seen in forty years of practice have been in those patients where the non-heroic, simple, ordinary intravenous fluid kept the patient alive during a week or more of stupor or coma, at the end of which time some consciousness returned but the patient was left with severe and totally incapacitating brain damage, no speech, no understanding, no bladder or bowel control.

There are a few exceptions, but by and large, if it takes intravenous fluids to keep you "alive" after a severe stroke, you are far better off dead!

No ethical doctor would or could ever make a unilateral decision not to use such ordinary means as intravenous fluids to keep a patient living, even though the coma or stupor went on for two weeks. The family too will refuse to "play God" and therefore it has to be the patient's decision. The patient must tell his doctor in advance, because the instant a devastating stroke has occurred, it is too late to communicate.

Your brain is the most easily damaged of all your vital organs. The older you are, the more easily it is damaged. Unlike a damaged liver, a damaged heart or kidney, a dead brain cell is never replaced by a new one.

In case I should have a stroke I have told my own doctor and my wife that if I am in a coma or a stupor, or if for any reason cannot communicate my wishes, there is to be no intravenous drip, no injection, no antibiotics, no cardiac monitoring, no cardiac pacing, no respiratory assistance, no tracheal intubation, no cerebral angiography, no resuscitation! If I cannot swallow solids, I can be offered clear liquids. If I cannot drink, I can be offered a teaspoon of water at frequent intervals. If I choke on that, the nurse can try a small ice chip. If my brain is so damaged that I cannot manage even that, so be it. But no intravenous fluids!

I far prefer, in the case of a severe stroke, to let the laws of the survival of the fit operate. I positively forbid any medical intervention. *Good nursing care* is all I will permit.

If I can survive with just good nursing care and no intravenous or antibiotics, I probably can be at least partially rehabilitated and will not be a nursing home candidate. If I survive only because of modern supportive medicine, I will in all probability be a vegetating burden to myself and my family, and society! *No, thank you!*

What if my own doctor was out of town when I was stricken and the doctor substituting for him should not agree to follow my instructions? My wife would replace him with a doctor who would understand my right, as clearly expressed in writing and duly witnessed, to decline *any type of treatment at any time for any reason that seems valid to me!*

As to the newly designed and established neurological intensive care units that would monitor ten bodily functions all at the same time, they might be helpful in a young person with a brain injured from a car accident, but for me, if I had a serious stroke, it would be unthinkable. My neurologist agrees with me.

Furthermore, I have discussed this strong belief of mine with many doctors over sixty and 90 percent agree with me that if they suffer a severe stroke, particularly a right-sided stroke in a right-handed person or a left-sided stroke in a left-handed person, and are stuporous or comatose and cannot swallow liquids or communicate their thoughts, they want absolutely no I.V. fluids started.

About 10 percent of the doctors I have spoken with approve intravenous fluids for one day, or they say, "Let my doctor and family decide."

I choose to err on the side of a quick death or a brief illness rather than hazard an unknowable degree of brain damage with my "survival" dependent on two days or two weeks of intravenous fluids.

A justly renowned American physician has committed himself publicly in this matter. Eugene Stead, M.D., Professor of Medicine at Duke University, wrote in a letter published in *Medical World News:*

> In case of a cerebral accident [stroke] other than a subarachnoid hemorrhage [a hemorrhage between the skull and the brain, *not* with the brain substance], *I want no treatment of any kind* until it is clear I will be able to think effectively. This means no stomach tubes and *no intravenous fluids.* [24]

## WHAT ABOUT CANCER?

Hans Zinsser, M.D., was a bacteriologist, author, philosopher, and poet. When he knew he was doomed to die of lymphatic leukemia (a cancer of white blood cells), he wrote a poem which has been of great philosophic benefit to many of my patients, some with cancer, some who dreaded it. It teaches the truth that in some older patients cancer should be looked upon as a possible friend who holds the sure promise of saving one from slow, senile disintegration and years in a so-called convalescent hospital.

Here is part of the poem:

> Now is death merciful. He calls me hence
>   Gently, with friendly soothing of my fears
> Of ugly age and feeble impotence
>   And cruel disintegration of slow years.
> Nor does he leap upon me unaware
>   Like some wild beast that hungers for its prey,
> But gives me kindly warning to prepare
>   Before I go . . .

He ends the poem:

> How good that ere the winter comes, I die![25]

Cancer should seldom lead to a nursing home. In the seventh, eighth, or ninth decades of life, cancer can be your friend.

About one third of all cancers are easily cured and therefore no problem.

A second third can be treated more or less effectively, giving an additional three to fifteen useful years of good *living*—not just existence.

A final third, at this stage in our knowledge, are fatal from the moment they begin, either because of their place of origin or the great malignancy of their cells.

One hundred years ago, Sir William Osler called pneumonia

"the old man's friend." Today it is almost impossible to die of pneumonia or any other infection, thanks to sulfa drugs, penicillin, and other antibiotics.

Therefore I tell my older patients who are afflicted with or fearful of incurable cancer that it can be a real friend. An advancing cancer, with death in a few weeks or months, has spared many an older patient years of increasing senility and institutionalization.

Fatal and progressing cancer can be cared for at home with the aid of a practical nurse and ample morphine or Demerol, a morphine derivative. Either drug can be taken by mouth and can control the patient's pain and discomfort for months. An advantage to being at home is that you don't have to wait for the nurse to bring your medicine. You can take as much as you need when you need it. You can even take it to prevent the onset of pain—not just to relieve it.

The majority of my patients who have died of cancer have done so at home with nursing assistance, or in a private hospital room for the last few days or weeks.

The hospice is excellent for the patient who has no family to give moral support and nursing assistance. A nursing home for the alert patient with cancer has the obvious drawbacks of being an institution where such a large percentage of the patients are disoriented and demented. A nursing home is only suitable for persons with terminal cancer which is so far advanced that they are generally unaware of the nature of their surroundings.

Fortunately, the progressive nature of terminal cancer is such that the patient's stay, even in a nursing home, will not be a long one.

I also advise my patients with progressing cancer to use morphine or Demerol taken by mouth for sleep and for rest, both physical and mental. Morphine is the best tranquilizer that has ever been discovered for a final illness. It is cheap, effective, and harmless.

## WHAT ABOUT ELECTIVE MAJOR SURGERY?

The only concern we have with elective major surgery in the patient over sixty-five is the rare cardiac arrest in the operating room. This instantaneously transforms a standard operative procedure into a catastrophic emergency fraught with the hazard of permanent brain damage. My position is that both my surgeon and my anesthesiologist would have to agree with me before surgery that an absolute maximum of a two-minute effort to resuscitate me be observed.

As for heroic emergency surgery with no opportunity to consider the pros and cons, I am opposed to it for myself, or for any of my patients over sixty-five. I far prefer a quick death to the questionable results of heroic surgery on an emergency basis such as is sometimes done for a large blood clot to the lung, for rupture of the main blood vessel in the abdomen, for a devastating hemorrhage between the brain and the skull, or heroic surgery following a severe car accident that caused multiple internal injuries and made me unable to partake in a carefully considered manner. But you have to decide for yourself. Don't wait! Ask your doctor the next time you see him what he thinks is best for you.

## WHAT ABOUT ADVANCING ILL HEALTH?

Every patient knows when his health is beginning truly to deteriorate and foreshadow a time when an extended care facility may loom up in the background.

The normal aging process is slow, nearly imperceptible. It is probably due, as Professor Jacques Monod postulates, to constantly occurring "quantum perturbations"[26] in the atomic structure of our DNA molecules, so that the new liver, bone, kidney, and heart cells produced in our seventh decade of life and after are defective and perform their functions less well. The process of aging is felt decade by decade, not week by week or month by month.

But advancing disease is clearly perceptible. It gives those who are willing to accept the warning ample opportunity not only to consult their doctor but to consult themselves. There is time for competent patients to reflect, ask questions, and decide how much or how little they want modern hospital medicine and surgery to *attempt* to do *for them* and *to them!*

Unless doctors know what a patient wishes, they may (with the best of intentions and even in the presence of progressive chronic illness) so order matters as to assure futile prolongation of the function of their patient's vital organs, for days, weeks, months, or years.

So, if you have a chronic progressing illness, other than cancer, and don't want to experience years of total invalidism or senility, you had better, while you are still capable of thinking clearly, make up your mind and tell your doctor and family what you want. It is my recommendation that you give positive direction that when you are unable to speak for yourself, you absolutely refuse *all* "routine" medicines, such as antibiotics, digitalis, and diuretics, which would simply prolong the process of your dying.

# Chapter 12

## The Patient
## Gives the Orders

> The advances of science have made the central question
> of modern medicine a moral one.
>
> William H. Baltzell, M.D., "The
> Dying Patient," *Archives of Internal
> Medicine,* January 1971

"In issues as basic as these, the patient must be the one who decides."[27] With these words of Robert M. Veach I am in complete agreement. Therefore, as commander in chief of your own person, it is your responsibility and your right to give your doctor *strategic* orders. You must supply him with specific guidelines reflecting your medical wishes should you have to be hospitalized for a serious illness.

Your doctor is well qualified to use all the medical tactics needed in the battle against a disease, but the doctor first needs to know *your* attitude toward aggressive or prolonged treatment.

In the absence of specific orders from you to the contrary, your doctor and the hospital are obliged by custom, law, and ethics to take every and all action, both routine and aggressive, necessary to prevent death and preserve your biological existence.

A unilateral decision by your doctor to do less than *every-*

*thing possible* to preserve the function of your vital organs is not permissible.

After you have carefully considered the matters presented in this book, it may be your desire to place specific limits on heroic treatment. You may decide that the general strategic approach to any serious illness you may suffer should be something less than all that the science and technology of medicine can now deliver. If so, you must, while you are well and sapient, give such specific orders to your doctor and make such orders available to any hospital in which you are likely to be a patient.

I do not propose to offer a blueprint for you to follow. Rather, I plan to outline the steps I have taken for myself to minimize the chances of spending the last years of my life in desuetude and despair in a nursing home.

These orders, in my belief, will protect me from having modern medical treatment exchange one fatal illness for another, leading thereby to invalidism, total dependence, and eventual institutional care.

I think the vast majority of doctors would feel deeply obliged to their patients over sixty-five for specifically indicating, in advance of any medical emergency, their well-considered strategic orders in regard to their own life and their own way of meeting death.

## THE RIGHT TO DIE

Right to Die laws have been passed in many states.[28] They all vary, but in general they only authorize the withholding or withdrawal of life-sustaining procedures for a patient with a *terminal* condition *who is of sound mind and voluntarily requests this to be done.*

None of the laws condone or authorize mercy killing nor permit any affirmative or deliberate attempt to end life.

Rather, the Right to Die laws permit the natural process of

dying and provide that this shall not for any purpose constitute a suicide.

Most laws require *formal certification by two physicians* that the patient is suffering from an incurable and terminal illness and that death is imminent, which usually means within a week or two.

It is true that the Right to Die laws make it a little easier now for your doctor to let you die from natural causes than heretofore.

However, they apply only to an *incurable and terminal illness* (this usually means cancer) from which it is expected that the patient will in any event die in less than two weeks. These laws do not help you avoid spending months or years in a nursing home from some chronic ailment that has been prolonged by medical measures to the point where you are totally unable lucidly to discuss the issues with your doctor.

In brief, the Right to Die laws do not directly address the slowly progressive, chronic, totally incapacitating medical diseases of the heart, kidneys, lungs, brain, and liver—the vital organs. Moreover, since these laws are only applicable in the terminal two weeks of your life, they are of no help in avoiding months or years in a convalescent hospital.

## HOSPITAL CONDITIONS OF ADMISSION

Before being admitted to a hospital, the patient must sign a document entitled Conditions of Admission. There is only one paragraph in this document that need concern you but it is an important one for you to consider. It usually reads something like this:

The patient hereby consents to the examinations, treatments, and medications ordered or recommended by the attending physician or any hospital medical staff physician designated by him.

This is, in reality, carte blanche authority for your doctor or any doctor on the medical staff called by him or the hospital to order any test or treatment which is, in his opinion, indicated. If you are alert, the doctor naturally will discuss the pros and cons of any such measure with you, and you could refuse any test or treatment that seemed questionable. But if you are so sick that you are unable to discuss the measures to be taken, the document that you, or some responsible person on your behalf, have signed on admission gives the doctor full permission to take charge of your person.

Therefore, if I were the patient being admitted to the hospital for a serious illness or major surgery, I would, in my own handwriting, alter the routine consent for care on the Conditions of Admission form. If I were too sick at the time of admission to do this, my wife or my adult children would do it for me, knowing my wishes.

Incidentally, my wife, who was recently admitted to the hospital for major surgery, was told by the admitting clerk that she could make no such alterations in the hospital Conditions of Admission form. I was with her and I asked the young lady at the admissions desk to refer the matter to the chief nurse, who immediately said that this was perfectly acceptable. The point of the anecdote is to remind you that hospital personnel are not as yet used to the patient giving orders.

I strongly recommend that any reader of this book who is over sixty-five and who is in general agreement with my point of view consider such an alteration. It is one specific way to retain some control over your own life or death in a crisis situation.

The opening paragraph of the usual form (which I consider far too broad and permissive) is as follows, with my own alteration in capital letters (the words I crossed out are in brackets):

## HOSPITAL CONDITIONS OF ADMISSION

1. *Consent for Hospital Care:*

IN STRICT ACCORDANCE WITH MY "MODIFIED LIV-ING WILL," I, _____, [The patient] hereby consent[s] to the examinations, treatments, and medications ordered or recommended by the attending physician or any _____ Hospital medical staff physician designated by him during the patient's stay in _____ Hospital.

## SURGEON'S AND ANESTHETIST'S PERMIT

I have the greatest respect for the skill and judgment of the surgeons and the anesthesiologists on our hospital staff and for the overwhelming majority of their colleagues throughout the country.

I trust them implicitly to perform any service for which I have signed my permission and whose pros and cons I have had time to consider carefully.

However, for a person of my age and beliefs, the unexpected and fortunately rare cardiac arrest during surgery needs, in my opinion, a special notation on the operating permit form which I must sign to conform to my own personal desires.

Here are excerpts from the usual form, showing my additions in capital letters:

### SURGEON'S AND ANESTHETIST'S PERMIT FOR OPERATION AND ADMINISTRATION OF ANESTHESIA

I, _____, authorize and direct _____ _____, M.D., my surgeon, and/or associates or assistants of his choice to perform the following operation: _____ _____ on me and/or to do any other therapeutic procedure that his or their judgment may dictate to be advisable for my well-being; the nature of the operation has been explained to me and no warranty of guarantee has been made as to the results or cure.

I hereby authorize and direct the above named surgeon and/or his associates or assistants to provide such additional services for me as he or they may deem reasonable and necessary, including, but not limited to, the administration and maintenance of the anesthesia, and I hereby consent thereto. IN CASE OF <u>CARDIAC ARREST</u> I PERMIT A <u>MAXIMUM</u> OF <u>TWO MINUTES*</u> ATTEMPT AT RESUSCITATION IF <u>INSTANTLY</u> DETECTED AND <u>IMMEDIATELY</u> TREATED.

Signed_____ (Relationship) _____
Witness_____ Date _____ Time _____

(A copy of this document is to be delivered to the patient)

*or FIVE MINUTES, if your doctor approves.


The most difficult moment in the life of a surgeon may well be when he has to walk through the heavy automatic doors leading from the surgery area to tell the waiting family of a patient who has been having routine elective surgery that the patient has just died on the operating table from a cardiac arrest. Every surgeon I know, faced with a sudden cardiopulmonary arrest during an operation, would direct heroic efforts to resuscitate the patient for no less than one half hour and perhaps for as long as an hour, if any hope to revive him remained.

Obviously, this is precisely what I am afraid of. As far as I am personally concerned, far better dead than demented from post-resuscitation brain damage.

If I am the patient and should be unfortunate enough to suffer a cardiopulmonary arrest in the operating room (which was instantly observed and treated), I would want my surgeon and my anesthetist to undertake all the standard resuscitation measures for *two minutes and absolutely no more,* as timed by the operating room clock. If within two minutes, spontaneous normal respiration and heartbeat were restored, I would consider the chances of my suffering brain damage practically nil. But I would ask my personal physician to leave orders in red (on my order sheet and in my progress notes) stating that I forbid resuscitation efforts for more than two minutes and if there should be a second arrest, I forbid further measures.

In fairness to my surgeon, he would have to be informed of this in advance and naturally would have to agree. If he did not agree, I would find a surgeon who did.

I am quite prepared to weigh the usual risk-benefit ratio of modern surgery. But I do not choose to accept even a 10 percent chance that a heroic, prolonged attempt at resuscitation in the operating room will find me awakening with a permanently damaged brain.

## PATIENT'S BILL OF RIGHTS

Many hospitals have copies of the patient's bill of rights in their admitting departments. Six states require this. Actually, the patient's bill of rights simply codifies good human relations and good hospital care. It restates the rights a patient has always had to refuse treatment of any kind and to have as full as possible an understanding of his medical condition.

As pointed out by Dr. Count D. Gibson, Jr., "Some doctors are offended by the patient's bill of rights. They feel it implies that the physician isn't an adequate guarantor of them." Dr. Gibson states that "most physicians see themselves as profoundly involved with their patients' interests."

Dr. Gibson then goes on to say that "the patient's bill of rights has no teeth" and "that if patients are going to lose rights, it will happen in a hospital."[29]

The patient's bill of rights probably serves a useful purpose in reminding doctors, nurses, and patients that the paternalistic attitudes of fifty years ago—that the doctor knows best—have to change with the scientific technical explosion. Therefore, medical and surgical morbidity—that is, illness and invalidism inadvertently caused by doctors—is a risk that hospital patients have to understand and to evaluate for themselves.

I think the patient's bill of rights has helped to make today's physician more aware of their patient's desire to fully participate in the crucial medical decisions that concern them, and it has encouraged some hospitalized patients to ask more searching and profound questions of their doctors.

But it is only effective if your doctor knows what you want and what you don't want from modern medical technology. *If* he knows this, your own doctor will guarantee your rights. Here is the patient's bill of rights as set forth by the American Hospital Association:

### PATIENT'S BILL OF RIGHTS

1. The patient has the right to considerate and respectful care.

2. The patient has the right to obtain from his physician complete current information concerning his diagnosis, treatment, and prognosis in terms the patient can be reasonably expected to understand. When it is not medically advisable to give such information to the patient, the information should be made available to an appropriate person in his behalf. He has the right to know, by name, the physician responsible for coordinating his care.

3. The patient has the right to receive from his physician information necessary to give informed consent prior to the start of any procedure and/or treatment. Except in emergencies, such information for informed consent should include but not necessarily be limited to the specific procedure and/or treatment, the medically significant risks involved, and the probable duration of incapacitation. Where medically significant alternatives for care or treatment exist, or when the patient requests information concerning medical alternatives, the patient has the right to such information. The patient also has the right to know the name of the person responsible for the procedures and/or treatment.

4. The patient has the right to refuse treatment to the extent permitted by law, and to be informed of the medical consequences of his action.

5. The patient has the right to every consideration of his privacy concerning his own medical care program. Case discussion, consultation, examination, and treatment are confidential and should be conducted discreetly. Those not directly involved in his care must have the permission of the patient to be present.

6. The patient has the right to expect that all communications and records pertaining to his care should be treated as confidential.

7. The patient has the right to expect that within its capacity a hospital must make reasonable response to the request of a patient for services. The hospital must provide evaluation, service, and/or referral as indicated by the urgency of the case. When medically permissible a patient may be transferred to another facility only after he has received complete information and explanation concerning the needs for and alternatives to such a transfer. The institution to which the patient is to be transferred must first have accepted the patient for transfer.

8. The patient has the right to obtain information as to any relationship of his hospital to other health care and educational institutions insofar as his care is concerned. The patient has the right to obtain information as to the existence of any professional relationships among individuals, by name, who are treating him.

9. The patient has the right to be advised if the hospital proposes to engage in or perform human experimentation affecting his care or treatment. The patient has the right to refuse to participate in such research projects.

10. The patient has the right to expect reasonable continuity of care. He has the right to know in advance what appointment times and physicians are available and where. The patient has the right to expect that the hospital will provide a mechanism whereby he is informed by his physician or a delegate of the

physician of the patient's continuing health care requirements following discharge.

11. The patient has the right to examine and receive an explanation of his bill regardless of source of payment.

12. The patient has the right to know what hospital rules and regulations apply to his conduct as a patient.

### "A LIVING WILL"

"A Living Will" is the most popular brochure in my office. More than 500,000 persons throughout America have signed this document.

"A Living Will," in my opinion, is well phrased for the young adult who is seriously injured in a car or motorcycle accident, or for the middle-aged patient whose general health is good and who suffers from a serious accident or illness.

*However, I do not think that the wording is sufficiently strong for a person of my age, with my beliefs.*

Furthermore, it is all too apt to "get lost" during the usual routine of having a patient admitted and treated in the hospital. It is likely to be overlooked by the doctors and the nurses called in an emergency.

As you will see from the Living Will reproduced below, I have made several modifications in mine. (My changes are shown in capital letters; the words I crossed out are in brackets.)

### A LIVING WILL

#### (PLACE ON FRONT OF MY HOSPITAL CHART)

*To My Family, My Physician, My Clergyman, My Lawyer—*

If the time comes when I can no longer take part in decisions for my own future, let this statement stand as the testament of my wishes:

If there is no [reasonable] VERY GOOD expectation of my MAK-
ING AN EXCELLENT recovery from physical or mental disability, I,_____, [request] DEMAND
that I be allowed to die and not be kept alive by artificial means or
heroic measures. Death is as much a reality as birth, growth, matu-
rity, and old age—it is the one certainty. I do not fear death as much
as I fear the indignity of deterioration, dependence, and hopeless
pain. I ask that drugs be mercifully administered to me for terminal
suffering even if they hasten the moment of death.

This request is made after careful consideration. Although this
document is not legally binding, you who care for me will, I hope,
feel morally bound to follow its mandate. I recognize that it places
a heavy burden of responsibility upon you, and it is with the intention of sharing that responsibility and of mitigating any feelings of
guilt that this statement is made.

NOTE: IN CASE OF CARDIAC ARREST WHICH IS
INSTANTLY DETECTED I PERMIT TWO MINUTES* MAX-
IMUM ATTEMPTS TO RESUSCITATE ME.

Date_____ Signed _____
Witnessed by: _____
　　　　　　　　 _____

*or FIVE MINUTES, if your doctor concurs.

On the top line I have printed "Place on front of my hospital chart," and I have underlined the words in red. This
will assure that on the usual hospital chart, which becomes
thicker and more difficult to peruse each day in the hospital,
this document which expresses *my orders* is in front, where
it will be seen.

In the second paragraph I have changed the word "reasonable" to "very good." A "reasonable expectation of my recovery" is open to many interpretations depending upon the philos-

ophy of the doctors and nurses. A "very good expectation" is more explicit.

I have also added the word "excellent," for if I am so desperately sick or seriously injured that I cannot discuss the matter with my doctors, I forbid measures to keep me alive in the hope of a possible recovery. I permit treatment in these circumstances only when there is a *very good* chance of an *excellent* recovery! An "excellent recovery" is specific; it says just what I mean.

In the next line I have changed the word "request" to "demand." I do not request that I be allowed to die. *I order that I be allowed to die* in the circumstances under discussion! I choose death rather than medicated existence!

Finally, you will see that I have written special "cardiac arrest" orders. These orders are similar to those written in a directive by Robert S. Morrison, M.D., of New York City, when he turned sixty-five. Many of my colleagues in their seventh decade of life whom I have personally quizzed have expressed similar views.

Our feeling is that after two minutes of attempted resuscitation, a sixty-five-year-old or older brain is too apt to be damaged by oxygen lack during the arrest to risk further attempts to restore respiration and a viable heartbeat.

Therefore these special cardiac arrest orders, which will be on the front of the chart, apply throughout my hospitalization whether I am on a coronary care unit, on the intensive care unit, in the emergency room, or in the operating room. The reason for absolutely forbidding attempted resuscitation if the cardiac arrest is not instantly observed is that in these circumstances no one knows how long the heart has stopped.

I have several copies of my modified Living Will on hand. My wife has a copy, my doctor has a copy, my adult children have copies, and my attorney has a copy. I carry one in my pocket notebook.

If I have to be hospitalized, either I or my wife will see that the admitting clerk has a copy to place on the front of my chart as well as an extra copy for the chief nurse on the floor to which I am assigned.

If there is to be surgery, my surgeon and my anesthetist will be given copies.

The modified Living Will permits a brief attempt at cardiopulmonary resuscitation. When this succeeds, it is a brilliant achievement which I would not wish to deny myself or my patients. But a prolonged attempt at resuscitation for a person my age is too often the means of exchanging a brief final illness for slow disintegration. The modified Living Will permits all recognized medical and surgical treatment so long as the patient who has signed it is able to discuss these matters lucidly with the physician. However, it specifically forbids routine existence-prolonging devices where the brain has been so badly damaged that the patient is unable to communicate any thoughts to the doctor.

I do not wish to awaken to find the reflective and language centers of my brain incapable of functioning while the more primitive parts of the brain which maintain respiration and heartbeat have been kept viable by a week or two of intravenous fluids.

The modified Living Will permits all recognized treatment of cancer. It only forbids the continuation of treatment when the patient is no longer able to communicate his wishes and his desires to the doctor.

Finally, the modified Living Will permits all major elective surgery and only forbids resuscitation following an arrest in the operating room for a period of time longer than two minutes.

If you and your doctor prefer less strongly worded *patient's orders,* the original Living Will may well suit you. The point is to encourage you to write *your* orders NOW!

## FOR THE OLDER PERSON LIVING ALONE

Many Americans in their seventh, eighth, or ninth decade of life live alone, some with families nearby, some without. These people are especially in danger of becoming, willy-nilly, caught up in the inexorable "hospital system" if some sudden catastrophe of a medical nature occurs in which they can no longer express their wishes.

For older persons living alone, I recommend that they have a copy of the modified Living Will in an envelope by their bedside and in an envelope by their telephone. I recommend that at all times they wear a Medic-Alert bracelet.

Thus, if a friendly neighbor calls the emergency ambulance for you because you have suffered a stroke and can't speak, documents stating your wishes are easily available for the emergency room doctors and nurses.

No system is infallible in this imperfect world. The recommendations I have made are the best that have yet come to my mind for the intelligent patient to *issue patient's orders* for a time when he or she may be unable for any reason to do so.


## NURSING HOME CONDITIONS OF ADMISSION

There is no perfect plan whereby any one of us may completely prevent the unhappy event of ending our life in a long-term-care institution.

Progressive senility in an older person whose vital organs still function, even without special medical treatment, but whose brain deteriorates because of aging blood vessels will always be a part of the human situation. Some of these people will have to be institutionalized.

But even for this kind of patient the number of weeks, months, or years of incarceration can be materially decreased. This can be done by stopping or by not starting the use of such routine existence-prolonging drugs as digitalis, powerful diuretics to get rid of fluid and edema, antibiotics for treating and preventing respiratory and urinary tract infections. These patients can be treated symptomatically to make them comfortable without being treated scientifically only to prolong their suffering.

I consider the usual Conditions of Nursing Home Admission form far too broad and permissive. Therefore, I recommend that now, while you are able, you execute a fail-safe directive to prevent the use of powerful drugs which only prolong your final act of dying. I have reproduced below my directive should I ever have to be admitted to a nursing home.

The following is from the usual Conditions of Nursing Home Admission form:

### CONDITIONS OF NURSING HOME ADMISSION

*Medical and Surgical Consent:* THE PATIENT IS UNDER THE CONTROL OF HIS ATTENDING PHYSICIANS and the facility is not liable for any act or omission in following the instructions of said physicians, AND THE UNDERSIGNED CONSENTS TO ANY MEDICAL TREATMENT OR SERVICES RENDERED THE PATIENT UNDER THE GENERAL AND SPECIAL INSTRUCTIONS OF THE PHYSICIAN.

I consider this *far* too broad and permissive. In place of it I suggest, with your doctor's approval, the following restrictive form which I have signed for myself:

### DIRECTIVE TO NURSING HOME AND RELEASE
*(To become part of any nursing home or convalescent hospital Admission Sheet or Conditions of Admission)*

Directive made this _____ day of (month) _____, (year) _____.
(name) I, _____, being of sound mind and voluntarily

wishing to make known my desires, do hereby declare:

If at some time in the future I am admitted to a nursing home, *and in the absence of my ability to give directions concerning my care,* it is my intention that this directive shall be honored by my family and physician(s) as the final expression of my legal right to refuse medical and surgical treatment and accept the consequences of such refusal.

I consent only to nursing care, pain medication, and needed sedation. NOTHING ELSE!

*All other medicines* of any type are STRICTLY FORBIDDEN!

I prohibit any type of medical or surgical treatment *UNDER ANY CIRCUMSTANCES!*

If I sustain a fracture or any other injury, I will allow sedation, *ample* and frequent pain medicine, immobilization, and ABSO-LUTELY NOTHING ELSE!

Diagnostic tests, except the required chest X-ray, ARE NOT PER-MITTED!

I may be assisted to drink, food may be offered, BUT SPOON-FEEDING IS FORBIDDEN!

Signed _____

The examples I have given of how I have modified the conditions for admission to a hospital or a nursing home, and the restrictions I have placed on the kind of treatment I will accept from a surgeon or anesthetist, may not express your desires. You may feel far less certain about what is best in your case than I do in mine. This is why I have insisted that you think about it while you can. Talk it over with your family and especially with your doctor. Relieve them of making decisions that you yourself can make better.

The major point I want to make is that it is right and proper for you to give the orders. It is your life, your suffering, and your death that we have been considering. It is only fitting that you should decide how you want to be treated.

# Concluding Observations

In our culture we find death an unpleasant subject to discuss. We avoid facing it as long as possible, but sooner or later it intrudes into the lives of all of us. Moreover, we know that inevitably we must all confront it. Because of our failure to be realists in regard to this most certain fact of life, death for increasing numbers has become a needlessly prolonged and agonizing ordeal.

I am convinced there is a better way to die than to vegetate in a nursing home or an extended care facility. There is no happy solution to the death dilemma, but there are approaches that are more acceptable than others.

As for me, if I am so seriously ill or injured that I am unable to participate lucidly in the surgical-medical decisions that affect my life, I choose to accept the benefits and risks of a natural death inherent in the many illnesses I may have to suffer after age sixty-five. In such circumstances I will avoid those medical measures which so often exchange a brief final illness for permanent brain damage or total invalidism and a lingering death in an institution.

I have stated my own convictions firmly and clearly. I do not offer them as the model that others must or even should follow. The dilemma I have described, however, is one we all must face, and if I have been successful in causing you to make some kind of informed decision in regard to your own life and death, my purpose will have been accomplished.

The late and renowned Thomas Huxley once said: "The Gods send me a swift and speedy end whenever my time comes. ... After all, that is the way to die, better a thousand times than drivelling off into eternity."[30]

# Afterword

Intellect distinguishes between the possible and the impossible; reason distinguishes between the sensible and the senseless; even the possible can be senseless.

> Max Born, cited in "The Dying
> Patient," *Archives of Internal
> Medicine,* January 1971

As a family doctor I have the highest regard for the overwhelming majority of my medical colleagues.

I respect their specialized knowledge and skill which surpasses mine in many fields.

My patients and I are grateful for the help we have received on many occasions from scores of consultants.

I hope that by strongly urging my readers to partake more actively in the important ethical decisions that involve their own life or death, I may be found to have been of help to all concerned.

# Notes

1. Henrik Ibsen, *Brand,* tr. by F. E. Garrett (E. P. Dutton & Co. Inc., 1915).

2. Norman Wentworth DeWitt, *Epicurus and His Philosophy* (University of Minnesota Press, 1954), p. 73.

3. Robert M. Veatch, *Death, Dying, and the Biological Revolution* (Yale University Press, 1976), p. 5.

4. *Ibid.,* pp. 18, 20.

5. Roland Stevens, M.D., *People's Weekly Magazine,* March 17, 1976.

6. Alexander Rush, M.D., *The Magazine of Rush—Presbyterian—St. Luke's Medical Center,* Vol. 9, No. 2 (Winter 1976–77), pp. 42–43.

7. Martin G. Netsky, M.D., cited in Charles Fried, LL.B. (Harvard Law School), "Terminating Life Support: Out of the Closet!" *The New England Journal of Medicine,* Aug. 12, 1976, p. 390.

8. Louis S. Baer, M.D., "Unloving Care," *The Western Journal of Medicine*, Vol. 127, pp. 338–339.

9. Maria Huxley, cited in Sybille Bedford, *Aldous Huxley: A*

*Biography* (Alfred A. Knopf, Inc., and Harper & Row, Publishers, Inc., 1974).

10. Hilaire Belloc, *Milton* (J. B. Lippincott Company, 1935).

11. Daniel Greenberg, M.D., in *The New England Journal of Medicine,* March 24, 1977, pp. 699–700.

12. Gunnar Biorck, M.D., "How Do You Want to Die?" *Archives of Internal Medicine,* October 1973, pp. 605–606.

13. W. T. Longcope, M.D., *Methods and Medicine,* Bulletin of Johns Hopkins Hospital, 1932.

14. Osler L. Peterson, M.D., "Evaluating Medical Technology," *Annals of Internal Medicine,* December 1976, p. 820.

15. Charles D. Aring, M.D., "Intimations of Mortality," *Annals of Internal Medicine,* July 1968, pp. 137–152.

16. The text of the following two cases has been edited only to omit much of the technical language.

17. Veatch, *Death, Dying, and the Biological Revolution.*

18. A phrase used by W. Keith Morgan, M.D., in a Letter to the Editor, *The New England Journal of Medicine,* Aug. 25, 1977, p. 456.

19. Pedro A. Poma, M.D., Mt. Sinai Hospital Medical Center of Chicago, Letter to the Editor, *The New England Journal of Medicine,* Aug. 25, 1977, p. 456.

20. J. W. Jacobs, M. R. Bernard, A. Depgada, *et al.,* "Screening for Organic Mental Syndromes in the Medically Ill," *Archives of Internal Medicine,* Jan. 1977, pp. 40–46.

21. Lillian Carter and Gloria Carter Spann, *Away from Home: Letters to My Family* (Simon & Schuster, Inc., 1977), p. 153.

22. Order forms and information available from Medic Alert Foundation International, Turlock, Calif. 95380. Phone: (209) 632–2371.

23. "Myocardial Infarction: Comparison Between Home and Hospital Care for Patients," *British Medical Journal,* April 17, 1976, pp. 925–928.

24. Eugene Stead, M.D., letter in *Medical World News,* April 7, 1972, p. 47, cited in Veatch, *Death, Dying, and the Biological Revolution,* p. 181.

25. Hans Zinsser, M.D., *As I Remember Him: The Biography of R. S.* (Little, Brown & Company, 1940).

26. Jacques Monod, *Chance and Necessity: An Essay on the Natural Philosophy of Modern Biology* (Vintage Books, 1972), p. 111.

27 Veatch, *Death, Dying, and the Biological Revolution,* p. 8.

28. Copies of the Right to Die laws may be obtained from the Euthanasia Council, 250 W. 57th St., New York, N.Y. 10019.

29. Count D. Gibson, M.D., in *The Stanford Observer,* Nov. 1977, p. 6.

30. Leonard Huxley, *Life and Letters of T. H. Huxley* (Appleton, 1900).